The Practical Approach to
Surgical Gastrointestinal and Hepatopancreatobiliary Diseases
A Clinical Handbook and Preparatory Manual

The Practical Approach to
Surgical Gastrointestinal and Hepatopancreatobiliary Diseases

A Clinical Handbook and Preparatory Manual

Advait Sanjay Sonar
MS(General Surgery), DrNB Surgical Gastroenterology(GI and HPB Surgery)
Postdoctoral Fellowship in GI Oncosurgery (Tata Memorial Hospital, Mumbai)
Fellow
Department of Surgical Oncology
HPB and UGI Unit
ACTREC, Tata Memorial Centre
Mumbai, Maharashtra, India

Forewords
Baiju Senadhipan
Shailesh V Shrikhande
M Kanagevel
Nissar Hussain Hamdani

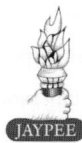

JAYPEE BROTHERS MEDICAL PUBLISHERS
The Health Sciences Publisher
New Delhi | London

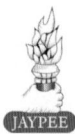 **Jaypee Brothers Medical Publishers (P) Ltd**

Headquarters
EMCA House
23/23-B, Ansari Road, Daryaganj
New Delhi 110 002, India
Landline: +91-11-23272143, +91-11-23272703
+91-11-23282021, +91-11-23245672
E-mail: jaypee@jaypeebrothers.com

Corporate Office
Jaypee Brothers Medical Publishers (P) Ltd.
4838/24, Ansari Road, Daryaganj
New Delhi 110 002, India
Phone: +91-11-43574357
Fax: +91-11-43574314
E-mail: jaypee@jaypeebrothers.com

Overseas Office
JP Medical Ltd.
83, Victoria Street, London
SW1H 0HW (UK)
Phone: +44-20 3170 8910
Fax: +44(0)20 3008 6180
E-mail: info@jpmedpub.com

Website: www.jaypeebrothers.com
Website: www.jaypeedigital.com

© 2025, Jaypee Brothers Medical Publishers

The views and opinions expressed in this book are solely those of the original contributor(s)/author(s) and do not necessarily represent those of editor(s) or publisher of the book.

All rights reserved. No part of this publication may be reproduced, stored or transmitted in any form or by any means, electronic, mechanical, photocopying, recording or otherwise, without the prior permission in writing of the publishers.

All brand names and product names used in this book are trade names, service marks, trademarks or registered trademarks of their respective owners. The publisher is not associated with any product or vendor mentioned in this book.

Medical knowledge and practice change constantly. This book is designed to provide accurate, authoritative information about the subject matter in question. However, readers are advised to check the most current information available on procedures included and check information from the manufacturer of each product to be administered, to verify the recommended dose, formula, method and duration of administration, adverse effects and contraindications. It is the responsibility of the practitioner to take all appropriate safety precautions. Neither the publisher nor the author(s)/editor(s) assume any liability for any injury and/or damage to persons or property arising from or related to use of material in this book.

This book is sold on the understanding that the publisher is not engaged in providing professional medical services. If such advice or services are required, the services of a competent medical professional should be sought.

Every effort has been made where necessary to contact holders of copyright to obtain permission to reproduce copyright material. If any have been inadvertently overlooked, the publisher will be pleased to make the necessary arrangements at the first opportunity.

Inquiries for bulk sales may be solicited at: jaypee@jaypeebrothers.com

The Practical Approach to Surgical Gastrointestinal and Hepatopancreatobiliary Diseases / Advait Sanjay Sonar

First Edition: **2025**

ISBN: 978-93-6616-624-7

Printed at: Sterling Graphics Pvt. Ltd.

DEDICATED TO

My parents (Sanjay and Swapna) and my aunt (Seema) who have always supported me in the difficult decisions that I have taken and my in-laws (Alpa and Yogesh) for always being supportive of my endeavors.

My wife (Shrusty) who has been there as a pillar of hope in some of the toughest times I went through and her unwavering patience, without whom I would have likely given up the thought of pursuing this field.

Foreword

"Whoever saves a single life, it is considered as if one saved the entire world."
—from the Talmud

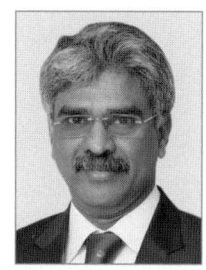

With the rapid expansion of surgical knowledge, it has never been more challenging to organize and articulate a simple and safe surgical plan. Traditional textbooks, in an attempt to keep pace with the growth of surgical science, have become encyclopedic reference books. Young surgeons, with a finite amount of time to pore over such tomes and an increasing load of clinical responsibilities, often search for educational materials that offer basic, safe principles of surgery. For the more seasoned surgeon, a brief review of vital surgical topics does not require the comprehensive perspective offered by traditional surgical textbooks. Dr Sonar created this book of surgical algorithms in order to meet the needs of both of these groups of surgeons. The goal of an algorithm is to create a set of rules, permit data processing, and establish a solution in the most efficient manner. An algorithmic approach to surgical scenarios allows for concise organization of clinical information, application of basic and safe principles, and, finally, formation of an unambiguous surgical solution. The algorithms are also accompanied with a synopsis to provide a more comprehensive review, if desired. Students, residents, and surgeons will find the algorithms concise enough to read to completion in moments of spare time. For the surgical trainee, they should provide a foundation upon which future learning can be built. At last this book provides must-know details about calories and electrolyte management necessary for surgeons.

Baiju Senadhipan
Professor
Founder, Senadhipan Education Foundation
Chairman and Managing Director
Senadhipan Institute of Medical Sciences
Thiruvananthapuram, Kerala, India

Foreword

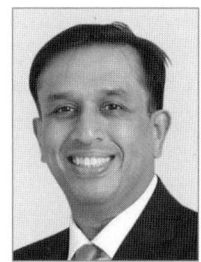

It is my pleasure to write a foreword for this book by my fellow Dr Advait Sonar. The book is pleasing to the eye. It is an excellent handbook and easy to refer and provides a comprehensive coverage of a broad range of topics that are commonly encountered cases in routine practice of surgical gastroenterology. The defining feature of this book is the amalgamation of specific history taking that is relevant to reaching a differential diagnosis that should ultimately guide necessary investigations in the run up to formulating a specific treatment approach. This aspect would be useful not just to the postgraduate and superspecialty students of surgery and surgical gastroenterology but also to the busy general surgeon who would value a quick update on modern-day surgical gastroenterology.

Last but not the least, I must congratulate Dr Sonar for conceiving the idea of this book so early in his surgical career. However, he has very clear reasons why he has chosen to do so. Having personally experienced the challenges and difficulties of residency and specialty examinations in surgical gastroenterology in his recent past, he has promptly embarked on this contribution with an aim to ensure that his younger colleagues have an easier path ahead negotiating the various twists and turns associated with residency that ultimately culminate in surgical gastroenterology examinations. This effort reflects the potential of a good-hearted teacher and will keep him in good stead in his journey ahead. I wish him the very best in his surgical career.

Shailesh V Shrikhande
MS(Mumbai) MD(Heidelberg) FRCS Eng(Ad Eundem) ASA(Hon)
FACS(Hon) FRCS Edin(Hon)
Deputy Director, Tata Memorial Hospital
Professor and Head, Division of Cancer Surgery
Chief, GI and HPB Service
Tata Memorial Centre
Mumbai, Maharashtra, India

Foreword

Friends and aspiring surgeons, I am happy to write a foreword for this unique publication meticulously authored by Dr Advait Sanjay Sonar.

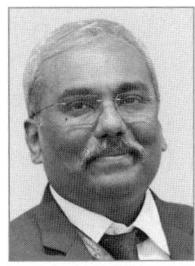

This book, *The "Practical" Approach to Surgical Gastrointestinal and Hepatopancreatobiliary Diseases*, focusing on a practical approach to gastrointestinal and hepatobiliary surgery promises a valuable resource for surgical trainees and practicing surgeons alike.

The wide array of contents suggests a well-structured approach, covering a broad range of common and complex surgical scenarios. The inclusion of ward management discussions alongside specific disease entities is a particularly welcome addition, as it bridges the gap between theoretical knowledge and real-world patient care. Important references are added to every topic as a ready reckoner and memory recall.

- Practical focus, comprehensive coverage, structured approach, emphasis on case presentation, and ward management integration are the stellar strengths of this book.
- *Depth of coverage*: While the breadth of topics is impressive, the depth of coverage within each chapter will be crucial to the book's overall value. A truly practical approach requires more than just a superficial overview; it needs to delve into the nuances of surgical techniques, decision-making, and potential complications.
- *Evidence-based approach*: A practical approach should ideally be grounded in evidence-based medicine. Thus, this book incorporates current research and guidelines to support its recommendations.

Overall: Based on a huge and unique collection of diverse topics, this book appears to be a promising addition to the surgical literature. Its focus on practical aspects, comprehensive coverage of GI and HPB conditions, and integration of ward management discussions are all positive features. The book's ultimate plus is the depth of coverage and its ability to translate theoretical knowledge into practical skills.

I am sure every reader will be benefited toward a better understanding and am sure the reader will have a much clearer outlook and focused approach toward examinations and management of gastrointestinal disorders.

I congratulate the author for this excellent publication.

M Kanagevel
DNB FRCS GI FACS FACRSI FALS FAGIE MMAS
Director Gastropro
Department of General, Gastrointestinal and Minimal Access Surgery
St. Isabel Hospital, Chennai, Tamil Nadu, India
Founder, National Postgraduate Surgical Clinics (YouTube Channel)
Founder, Evidence-based Surgery (Social Media)

Foreword

It is a rare and special honor to introduce the work of my student who has embarked on the journey of authoring a book. This book, I know, has been crafted in thoughts much before it actually took its physical form.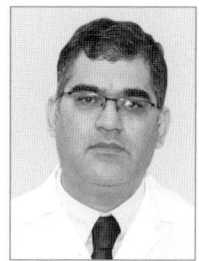

The primary aim of writing this book, as Dr Advait Sanjay Sonar shared many times with me, was the urge to condense the knowledge of the timeless pearls of great teachers in the field of gastrointestinal (GI) and hepatopancreatobiliary (HPB) surgery who have devoted themselves to the education and training new generations of GI and HPB surgeons for students who are less privileged.

This book is primarily meant for the students who are preparing for outgoing postdoctoral practical exams in the specialties of surgical GI, GI and HPB surgical oncology, and general surgery residents. Every idea within these pages reflects a unique case scenario and the approach one needs toward it.

As a teacher, I have had the privilege of witnessing the growth of the author Dr Advait Sanjay Sonar—not just as a writer but as a clinician and as a surgeon. I wish this literary endeavor of Dr Advait Sanjay Sonar be one of the many projects he undertakes in his life. I wish him success and contentment in serving his patients and teaching his students. May this book be the first of many accomplishments in your journey. May he achieve the success of both heart and mind.

With pride and admiration,

Nissar Hussain Hamdani
Professor and Head
Department of Surgical Gastroenterology (GI and HPB Surgery)
Government Medical College
Srinagar, Jammu and Kashmir, India

Preface

The "Practical" Approach to Surgical Gastrointestinal and Hepatopancreatobiliary Diseases is exactly what it purports to be: How your approach to exams and also in clinical decision-making must be.

Why this book?

I realized that there were a multitude of books which focused on the preliminary part of case presentation, but none of them addressed how to actually approach a case practically, starting from diagnosis and summary, leading to the management, which was expected of a candidate by gastrointestinal (GI) surgery examiners.

During the exam, after the differential diagnoses, examiners ask how you want to proceed. So this has two aspects, one is the sequence of the tests you want to do, which must be backed by a sound logic, and the other is the treatment part.

This book comprehensively covers all of this, including the latest studies/trials which I have mentioned in the management part of a particular topic and also toward the end.

But keep in mind that this field is rapidly advancing, and hence, the latest literature must be referred to, before any exam.

Along with this, TNM staging has been included toward the end of the book for easy referral.

How to use?

- This book's primary focus will be on how to approach a case comprehensively management wise, along with clinical tips along the way.
- Thinking retrospectively, this book will help you right from the start of your surgical residency, theory exams, clinical exams as well as in your clinical practice!
- The first chapter is a primer for all cases. It will give you tips for clinical examination in a GI and hepatopancreatobiliary (HPB) case.
- The rest of the chapters are about the most common cases which will be given to you in your examination, which include history and examination followed by management of the particular case followed by the "ward" section which includes the most common postoperative complications and their management.
- All of the discussions in this book are influenced by the approaches taken by premier surgical institutes in the country to these complex cases/situations.

Who will benefit?

- Superspeciality residents (those pursuing their doctoral degree in Surgical Gastroenterology and Surgical Oncology) all over India for their exit exams
- Superspeciality aspirants (Surgical Gastroenterology and Surgical Oncology)

- General Surgery Residents (Postgraduates)
- Budding clinicians/practising general surgeons

Now let me break down each of these groups:
- **Superspeciality exit exam (for Surgical Gastroenterology and Surgical Oncology):**
  - Superspeciality degree is for 3 years and the exit exam is held at the end of the academic course.
  - It is the toughest exam to crack, which is quite a challenge to pass, especially the national board (DrNB) exit.

Reasons for this are:
⇨ Surgical Gastroenterology and Surgical Oncology are highly coveted superspeciality fields; as a result, the examiners for the exit exams allow little room for error.
⇨ The theory exam tests your knowledge, but the practical exam is a different beast. Along with the knowledge, you need to know how to actually manage a patient, how to investigate, and what decision to take in a particular situation.

So how does this exam work: The candidate needs to pass the theory exam, after which he/she becomes eligible for the practical exam. If the candidate fails the practical exam in the first attempt, he/she is allowed to reappear after 6 months. If the candidate fails again, then he/she has to reappear for the theory exams.

How does the practical exam go about?
The exam is divided into 3 parts:
1. Four long cases
2. Ward rounds
3. Table viva (instruments, recent trials, procedures)

Of these, the long cases and the ward rounds form the major chunk of the candidate's marks. This decides whether he/she will be passed or not.

There are 3–4 candidates/session. The exam begins in the morning and generally goes on till evening (the candidate's performance and the examiner's irritation are indirectly and directly proportional, respectively, to the duration of the exam).

The long cases and ward rounds are the first to be taken, followed by the table viva.

How does a long case proceed?
Each candidate is allotted 30–45 minutes for the case, in which he/she has to complete the following:
- History
- Examination
- Writing the summary of the case
- Listing the differential diagnoses

After this, the candidate is summoned to the interrogation room to present his/her case.

Depending upon the mood of the examiner, the candidate may be asked to go sequentially from history to differentials, or the examiner may just ask point-blank to summarize the case and give the differentials.

Thus, writing a crisp summary and listing the relevant differentials (possible and not just probable) are the key to happiness (of both the candidate and the examiner).

Once the preliminaries are done, the examiner will ask:
How do you want to proceed?

Now this is the heart and brain of your exam. This part of the exam (the management of a case) will make or break your day, which is the reason for the candidates' dismal pass rates.

So here you will tell the examiner how you want to investigate the patient.

Now this is very important, as the examiner will ask you why you want to order a certain investigation and why not an alternate one. If you defend yourself, you get the marks for it. If you do not, then you will lose marks for it.

After this, you will be asked your final diagnosis.

If you ace this part, then the examiner will proceed with the actual management of the case (surgery/chemotherapy/observation and the latest studies).

This is followed by postoperative ward rounds. You will be told what procedure the patient has undergone and then you will be asked questions regarding the management of the case and complications of the procedure (your day-to-day management of ward during the 3 years of your residency, along with the "ward" section from this book, is all that you need to crack this part).

This will be followed by the table viva.

- **Superspeciality aspirants (Surgical Gastroenterology and Surgical Oncology)**, i.e., those who are preparing for national entrance exams, as a reference book, as many questions asked in the entrance are based on clinical situations.
- **General surgery residents (Postgraduates):** For those who want an in-depth knowledge of core GI and HPB clinical management.
- **Budding clinicians/practising general surgeons,** who will benefit in decision-making, as such complicated cases are often encountered by them in their OPDs, and knowing the proper management will help them as well as their patients.

Advait Sanjay Sonar

Acknowledgments

I wish to sincerely thank the innumerable teachers and seniors in the field of Gastrointestinal (GI) and Hepatopancreatobiliary (HPB) surgery, many of whom I have not met personally, but whose teachings reached directly or indirectly to us through their lectures, books, research papers, and online platforms. These have been a source of priceless and distilled knowledge for me and for my colleagues all over India, when we were preparing for our Surgical Gastroenterology/GI and HPB Oncosurgery exit exams and even now, when we are practising GI and HPB surgeons ourselves.

I specifically want to thank:
- Professor (Dr) Vinay K Kapoor and his team, for organizing online, Jaipur Surgical Tutorials, which made it possible for students like me to have access to the best national faculty including him, from whom I have learned so much during my exam preparation and continue to do so.
- Professor (Dr) Pradeep Rebala, for organizing online "Monday clinics", which include teachings from Pan-India GI and HPB surgical faculty of the highest order.
- Professor (Dr) Puneet Dhar, for organizing National Board of Examination's online Friday clinics, from which I have learned immensely.
- Professor (Dr) Baiju Senadhipan, for organizing the "Senadhipan Education Foundation" academic sessions which provide an access to the teachings from the best national and international faculty in GI and HPB surgery, from which I have learned so much and continue to do so.

I wish to sincerely thank Jaypee Brothers Medical Publishers for publishing the book and for being always available to discuss new ideas for the same.

I am forever indebted to my loving family, all my teachers, and my patients, without whom all of this would be pointless.

Last but not the least, I want to thank my professors at the Department of Surgical Gastroenterology (GI and HPB Oncosurgery), Superspeciality Hospital, Government Medical College, Srinagar and my professors at the Department of GI Surgical Oncology, Tata Memorial Hospital and at ACTREC, Tata Memorial Centre, Mumbai, whose active clinical discussions during ward rounds, outpatient work, and even while operating upon our patients paved the way for this humble beginning.

Advait Sanjay Sonar

Contents

1. Few Tips for Overall Case Presentation — 1
2.1. Upper Gastrointestinal—Esophagus and Stomach Cases — 5
2.2. Upper Gastrointestinal—Corrosive Injury — 35
2.3. Upper Gastrointestinal—Ward — 47
3.1. Hepatopancreatobiliary: Malignant Surgical Obstructive Jaundice—History/Examination Discussion — 53
3.2. Hepatopancreatobiliary—Surgical Obstructive Jaundice Approach — 61
3.3. Hepatopancreatobiliary—Management of Cases besides Gallbladder Cancer — 65
3.4. Hepatopancreatobiliary—Gallbladder Cancer Management — 85
3.5. Hepatopancreatobiliary—Imaging Lesions — 91
3.6. Hepatopancreatobiliary—Ward — 97
4. Bile Duct Injury — 107
5. Chronic Pancreatitis — 115
6. Non-cirrhotic Portal Hypertension — 131
7.1. Colorectal—Rectal Prolapse and Cancer — 145
7.2. Colorectal—Inflammatory Bowel Disease and Intestinal TB — 164
7.3. Colorectal—Ward — 176
8. Lump in Abdomen — 178
9. Electrolytes and Calories in Two Minutes — 191
10. TNM Staging of Gastrointestinal and Hepatopancreatobiliary Cancers — 193
11. Clinical Trials — 202

Index — 215

CHAPTER 1

Few Tips for Overall Case Presentation

REMEMBER

■ IN HISTORY PART OF CASE PRESENTATION

- Positive history to be recorded in patient's words only.
- Negative history to be recorded in medical terms only.
  (So if he says bloody vomiting, mention it as it is. But if it's part of negative history, then mention it as: no history of hematemesis)

■ IN EXAMINATION PART OF CASE PRESENTATION

- Everything to be recorded in medical terms. Remember to follow the proforma of—General examination, Abdominal examination and then Systemic examination.
- Remember to do a complete per rectal examination in all cases and a detailed respiratory system examination in cases of ailments of the esophagus.

■ IN SUMMARY PART OF CASE PRESENTATION

All positive history again to be recorded in patient's words only. Rest of all to be recorded in medical terms. Mention negative history, only if it is very significant, otherwise mention only positive history. Whereas in examination part of summary, mention all the positive findings first, and after that if everything else was noncontributory, you can say that rest of the examination is unremarkable.

■ HOW TO WRITE SUMMARY OF THE CASE

At times, when examiners are tired of listening to students drone on and on about history and examination, they may ask you upfront to directly present the summary of your case. Hence, writing a concise and precise summary is golden.

How to Formulate Summary

Though in history taking we start from age, sex, residence, occupation, etc., and after that come to the history of presenting illness (HOPI), positive and negative history, and then finally to treatment, past, personal, family and performance history, this sequence has to be altered for presenting the summary.

So begin with age, sex, residence [only if significant, like in case of gallbladder cancer (GBC) which has a high incidence in North India, while chronic pancreatitis (CP) has a high incidence in Kerala, and Odisha], occupation/school class [only to show how the quality of life is being affected, like in CP with disabling pain and in extrahepatic portal vein obstruction (EHPVO) to show poor scholastic performance], then mention about comorbidities (such as DM, HTN, etc.) followed by performance status (as per WHO/ECOG score). Then taking a 180° turn, go in this order: Personal, Past, Family history, HOPI, precise positive history, relevant negative history (like no history of domiciliary birth/umbilical sepsis in a case of EHPVO), status (meaning whatever treatment patient has received till now), followed by positive and negative examination findings [only if relevant—like no stigmata of chronic liver disease in a case of portal hypertension to differentiate between chronic liver disease and noncirrhotic portal hypertension (NCPH)].

■ HOW TO ARRIVE AT A DIAGNOSIS AND HOW MANY DIFFERENTIAL DIAGNOSES (DDs) TO MENTION

Majority of the times, the history and examination (H/E) will lead you to a diagnosis. Do not mention more than three DDs as it may lead you astray.

When H/E is regarding a lump in abdomen, but it is not specific to any particular pathology, say that at present I am not able to reach a diagnosis, but based on the H/E and the site of the lump, I would like to keep benign/malignant DDs arising from so and so organs (in that area).

When H/E are completely inconclusive, say that I am not able to reach a diagnosis at present and would like to investigate the patient further.

In cases with a prolonged history, e.g., ulcerative colitis (UC) since 8 years [or any pathology with a protracted course of presentation and multiple treatments, spanning years like CP, or oriental cholangiohepatitis (OCH) or any case with related HOPI and chief complaints], write in chief complaints: what actual complaint he came with now to the hospital (e.g., pain in abdomen since 1 week). After that in HOPI, say that his/her history dates to 8 years back, and start from 8 years ago, including relevant negative history and treatment received as per chronology, and keep repeating this pattern for every episode, till you come to the chief complaints of present time, and then finally mention HOPI of the present chief complaints, again including relevant negative history and treatment history of this time, followed by the usual proforma up to examination.

For all other cases with unrelated past history, HOPI will strictly be about chief complaints only, and the unrelated history will come later as part of past history.

If symptoms are vague, like epigastric pain/bloody vomiting, etc., and even examination is unremarkable, then say that, at this moment I am not able to come to a diagnosis, but considering the site of pain (epigastric) and associated symptoms, I would like to consider in my DDs benign pathology (if the history suggests) or malignancy (if the history suggests) arising from stomach, liver, gallbladder, pancreas and retroperitoneal region, transverse colon, and further evaluate my patient.

Now, only if probed to give a specific diagnosis, then give a specific diagnosis. So if history is suggesting benign pathology, give all possible benign DDs originating from each of the above possible organs. And if it is suggesting a malignant pathology, then give all possible malignant DDs originating from each possible organ. Also if more likely benign but malignancy is a possibility, mention it only toward the end.

For all cases, say, You want to review all previous blood investigations, viral serology (routine workup), USG abdomen and pelvis, Chest X-ray (CXR), CECT (contrast-enhanced computed tomography), MR, ERCP (endoscopic retrograde cholangiopancreatography) and any biopsy, UGIE (upper gastrointestinal endoscopy) and any biopsy and any previous operation records.

Just remember while reading imaging, to please mention all negative findings as well, not just the positive ones, because they are as important.

Speak out everything that you know.

Then say I want to get two sets of investigations: one to aid/confirm diagnosis and stage the disease, and the other to complete the workup of the patient. (including cardiorespiratory and endocrine workup after diagnosis is complete and treatment plan is made).

Now for diagnosis of a likely luminal case, if patient is stable, then ask for UGIE/LGIE with biopsy first, and follow-up with USG abdomen and pelvis, CXR and other imaging, because first priority is to get the definitive diagnosis.

But if patient is unstable/presenting with bleed/vomiting, then first hemogram, electrolytes, KFT are essential, because if Hb is low then you need to build up Hb first, electrolytes need to be corrected, and only then shift for UGIE/LGIE after stabilizing.

For hepatopancreatobiliary (HPB) cases, first ask for USG abdomen and pelvis, and CXR to rule out distant metastases. If negative, only then proceed with the rest of the investigations.

At the end of all investigations, when you have decided what the plan is, remember all that you normally do, to prepare a patient in your ward.

■ SO FOR PREOPERATIVE FITNESS AND PLAN

- Cardiopulmonary evaluation including ECG, 2D echo, PFT, physician consultation for optimization of patients comorbidities (cardiorespiratory, asthma, BP, sugar, etc.) and reviewing medication, nutritional optimization, chest physiotherapy (prehabilitation).
- Preanesthesia checkup (PAC) to be done for risk assessment.

- MultiDisciplinary Tumor board (MDT) discussion and detailed counseling before chemo/surgery.

FEW DAYS BEFORE SURGERY

- Special preparation like nasogastric tube decompression and saline washes for gastric outlet obstruction (GOO), 2–3 days prior to surgery.
- Liquid diet followed by Mechanical bowel preparation (MBP) with oral antibiotics along with stoma site marking for colorectal cases.
- Adequate hydration, vitamin K for at least 3 days, fresh frozen plasma (FFP)/cryo for surgical obstructive jaundice (SOJ).
- Vaccination [Pneumococcal, *Haemophilus influenzae* type b (Hib), Meningococcal] 2 weeks prior to anticipated splenectomy.

JUST THE DAY BEFORE SURGERY

- Take consent, keep blood products ready, injection TT to be administered, then on morning of surgery advised patient to take bath with antiseptic followed by nasal mupirocin for MRSA (Methicillin-resistant *Staphylococcus aureus*) carriers.
- Deep vein thrombosis (DVT) prophylaxis with stockings/pneumatic compression and low-molecular-weight heparin (LMWH) 12 hours prior.
- Antibiotics given IV 1 hour before skin incision and then skin preparation done on table after induction.

MEDICATION

- Continue steroids, anti-HTN on day of surgery, withhold morning dose of insulin/oral hypoglycemic agent (OHA). Give aspirin upto the day before.
- Warfarin to be changed to UFH/LMWH 2 weeks prior to surgery, and can be continued up to 6 and 12 hours prior to surgery respectively.
- Stop newer direct oral anticoagulants 24–48 hours before.
- Stop clopidogrel 5 days before.

CHAPTER 2.1

Upper Gastrointestinal—Esophagus and Stomach Cases

■ HISTORY AND EXAMINATION IN A CASE OF DYSPHAGIA

Due to following three main differentials:
1. Esophageal cancer
2. Gastroesophageal junction (GEJ) cancer (esophageal/proximal stomach)
3. Achalasia

■ HISTORY OF DYSPHAGIA (DIFFICULTY IN SWALLOWING)

Transfer Dysphagia

Difficulty in transferring food from oral cavity into the esophagus via the pharynx. History of difficulty initiating swallowing, choking or coughing within first few seconds after swallowing food, nasal regurgitation, nasal twang, dysarthria: suggests oropharyngeal/transfer dysphagia etiology being neurological cause like neurovascular event.

Remember that, *short duration odynophagia* (pain during swallowing) is seen with tonsillitis/pharyngitis/retropharyngeal abscess and immediately after corrosive ingestion.

History of halitosis, neck swelling, gurgling sound along with neck swelling—most probably Zenker's diverticulum.

Esophageal Dysphagia

Old age, short history of dysphagia, which is painless progressive from solids to liquids, with loss of appetite and significant weight loss points to malignant cause of dysphagia.

So for short history of painless progressive dysphagia (etiology most likely to be malignant):
- Esophageal cancer
- GEJ cancer
- Proximal stomach cancer

But generally young age, long history of intermittent dysphagia (which may become progressive in achalasia) to liquids first or to liquids and solids equally, associated with chest pain, regurgitation, and there may be weight loss due to food fear *but no loss of appetite or* long history of stable/progressive painless dysphagia, with multiple endoscopic interventions points to benign cause of dysphagia.

Long history of intermittent dysphagia (likely benign causes) and often associated with pain after swallowing:
- Achalasia (long history starting with intermittent dysphagia to liquids then even solids, which becomes progressive in nature)
- Distal esophageal spasm (DES)/hypercontractile esophagus
- Esophagitis (stasis, reflux, eosinophilic, viral, fungal)

Long duration stable dysphagia:
1. Webs and rings (postcricoid webs seen in Plummer–Vinson, Schatzki ring seen with hiatus hernia in lower esophagus)
2. Peptic stricture (with history of GERD)

Long history of progressive dysphagia:
1. Achalasia
2. Corrosive strictures

Grade

Modified Takita's grading of dysphagia:
- *Grade 1*: Able to swallow solid meals
- *Grade 2*: Needs liquids to swallow solid meals
- *Grade 3*: Able to swallow only semisolids
- *Grade 4*: Able to swallow liquids alone
- *Grade 5*: Able to swallow saliva alone
- *Grade 6*: Unable to swallow even saliva
  Mention the progression to present grade.

Take the following history as well, in a case of dysphagia:
- *Site of food getting stuck neck/upper chest/lower chest*: Actual site of obstruction is below the site of obstruction as perceived by the patient.
- *History of associated sudden gripping band like chest pain (after having swallowed the food bolus) with dysphagia* generally more to liquids suggests motility disorder
- *History of dysphagia resulting due to consumption of hot or cold beverages*: Points more toward motility disorder.
- *History of postural modulation to facilitate swallowing*: Some patient extend their neck and/or straighten their spine to facilitate the act of swallowing. It is usually seen in long-standing dysphagia of benign etiology as in motility disorder.
- *History of regurgitation*: Motility disorder or gastroesophageal reflux disease (GERD)

- *History of long-standing GERD (heartburn, regurgitation)*: Suspect peptic stricture/GEJ cancer
- *History of corrosive intake*: To rule out dysphagia secondary to esophageal stricture.
- *History of aspiration pneumonitis*: Secondary to aspiration of food due to stasis of food due to progressive esophageal obstruction which is seen with achalasia cardia and corrosive injury
- *History of hematemesis/melena*: Due to tumoral bleed or rarely in severe acute corrosive injury. Remember that multiple endoscopic interventions for variceal bleed especially sclerotherapy may lead to dysphagia.
- *History of advanced unresectable esophageal malignancy*
- *History of hoarseness of voice*: Recurrent laryngeal nerve involvement
- *History of choking or coughing after swallowing food—Ono's sign*: Points toward tracheoesophageal fistula.
- *History of back pain and recent nontraumatic fractures*: Points toward malignancy involving posterior mediastinal nerve roots/vertebrae
- *History of loss of weight (LOW), loss of appetite (LOA)*:
  - Beware: Loss of weight happens in benign (corrosive stricture, achalasia) as well as malignant causes, however LOA happens with malignancy only
- *History of metastatic disease*:
  - Abdominal distension: Due to malignant ascites
  - Dry cough, hemoptysis: Due to pleural effusion and lung metastasis
  - Bony pain, nontraumatic fractures: Due to bony metastasis
  - Back pain: Due to to vertebral metastasis
  - Unexplained sudden new onset headaches, blackouts, seizures: Due to brain metastasis
- *Treatment history* of having undergone endoscopy, biopsy, administration of chemotherapy, radiotherapy points towards diagnosis of malignant dysphagia. Remember that achalasia, webs and rings, peptic stricture and corrosive strictures have history of multiple endoscopic interventions.
- *Past history*:
  - Past history of oral or upper digestive tract cancer: Higher risk for esophageal cancer due to field cancerization (SCC)
  - History of comorbid illness: Especially bronchial asthma and COPD which need extensive respiratory optimization before surgery
- *Personal history*:
  - Smoking history: As an etiology for malignancy and in anticipation of delayed weaning off ventilator and delayed wound healing
- *Performance history*:
  - As per ECOG (Eastern Cooperative Oncology Group) classification to know if the patient will tolerate surgical stress or at least chemo/radiotherapy.

ECOG Performance Score

0: Fully active, no performance restriction
1: Fully ambulatory and able to carry out light work. Strenuous physical activity restricted

2: Capable of all self-care but unable to carry out any other work activities. Up and about >50% of waking hours
3: Capable of only limited self-care, confined to bed or chair > 50% of waking hours
4: Completely disabled, cannot carry out any self-care; totally confined to bed/chair

■ EXAMINATION PROFORMA

General Examination: Part A
- *Visual appearance*:
  - Young/middle aged/elderly
- *Gender*:
  - Male/female
- *Built*: Poor/average/good
- *Nourishment*: Poor/average/good
- *Poor nourishment features*:
  - Temporal wasting
  - Sunken eyes
  - Flattened cheeks, Buccal hollow
  - Supraclavicular hollow
  - Squaring of shoulders
  - Prominent scapula
  - Prominent intercostal spaces
  - Scaphoid abdomen
  - Prominent hip bones
  - Prominent knee and elbows
  - Pedal edema
  - Decreased mid arm circumference
  - Decreased skinfold thickness
  - Measure height, weight, BMI
- *Clinical evaluation*:
  - Conscious/stuporous
  - Cooperative/uncooperative
  - Orientation to time, place and person: Present/absent
  - Hydration status: Hydrated/dehydrated
  - Lying comfortably bed/in discomfort/in pain
  - Whether patient prefers sitting or lying down position
  - Febrile/Afebrile
  - Vitals: Pulse, BP, respiratory rate, mention performance status here as well

General Examination: Part B
- *Look for PICCLE*: Pallor, icterus, cyanosis, clubbing, generalized or localized lymphadenopathy, palpable cervical and left supraclavicular lymph node, pedal or dependent edema

- *Examination of oral cavity.*
  Look for:
    - Mouth opening: Reduced mouth opening/trismus signifies submucosal fibrosis (can lead to upper digestive tract SCC) or oral malignancy
    - Mucosal lesion: Leukoplakia, erythroplakia, ulcers or growth. Esophageal cancer may occur many years after patient has been subjected to radiotherapy for HFN malignancies
    - Tongue movement: Restricted tongue movement points toward local tumor infiltration or neurovascular event which may have happened
    - Foul smell/halitosis: Seen with Zenkers, achalasia, corrosive strictures

Abdominal Examination

- *Look for* the presence of any feeding jejunostomy (FJ) which may be done for feeding access in cases of complete dysphagia.
- *On inspection, see if:*
    - Abdominal contour: Flat/distended/scaphoid
    - Umbilicus: Central/displaced. Inverted/everted/flat
    - All quadrants are moving equally with respiration or not
    - Any visible lump/nodule

  Look for: Visible scar, sinus, engorged veins, pulsations, peristalsis or cough impulse:
    - Inspect the groin hernial sites and examine genitalia.
    - Inspection of renal angles to look for fullness
- *On palpation, see if:*
    - Abdomen is soft, nontender
    - Liver is palpable or not (hepatomegaly may be present in case of liver metastasis)
    - If palpable, measure its extent from costal margin in midclavicular line

  See if:
    - It is tender/nontender
    - Consistency is soft/firm/hard
    - Surface is smooth/nodular
    - Borders are round/sharp, regular/irregular
    - Margins
    - Spleen is enlarged or not

  Look for umbilical nodule/Sister Mary Joseph nodule which would suggest disseminated disease:
    - Palpate groin hernia sites and examine genitals

  Look for tenderness in renal angles:
    - Examine back and spine for tenderness.
- *On percussion:*
    - Look for upper border of liver dullness (generally in the 5th intercostal space) in midclavicular line
    - Note the liver span (normal being 12–14 cm)

  Percussion note in the rest of the abdomen (generally tympanic)
  Tests for free fluid

- *On auscultation*:
  - Auscultate for bowel sounds.
  - Bruit, hum and rub
- *Per-rectal examination*: Look for metastatic deposits in the pouch of Douglas (Blumer Shelf)

Respiratory Examination

- *Inspection*:
  - Tracheal position: Midline/deviated
  - Bilateral chest movement: Equal or not
- *Palpation*:
  - Trachea central or deviated
  - Bilateral chest movement: Equal or not
  - Chest, look for warmth and tenderness
  - Tactile vocal fremitus: It is increased in case of pleural effusion and consolidation.
- *Percussion*:
  - Normal percussion note is resonant.
  - Dull note suggests consolidation or pleural effusion.
- *Auscultation*:
  - Breath sounds
  - Bilaterally equal or not
  - Reduced breath sounds would suggest either pleural effusion or consolidation
- *Adventitious sounds*:
  - Crepts: Coarse crepts would suggest aspiration pneumonitis, whereas fine crepts would suggest pulmonary edema.
  - Rhonchi/Wheeze

So just remember that increased tactile vocal fremitus (TVF) on palpation, a dull-note on percussion and reduced breath sounds on auscultation point toward pleural effusion/lung consolidation.

Rest of the systemic examination

■ HISTORY AND EXAMINATION IN A CASE OF GASTRIC OUTLET OBSTRUCTION

It is most often seen due to stomach cancer/lymphoma/peptic/corrosive stricture.
- *History of pain*: Points toward malignant transformation of gastric peptic ulcer. Pain of gastric peptic ulcer is in the epigastrium, dull in nature, precipitated by meals, whereas pain in duodenal ulcer is precipitated by fasting, may radiate to back and is relieved on consuming meals and duodenal ulcer does not turn malignant.
- *History of dyspepsia*: Long-standing dyspepsia points toward peptic ulcer, which may progress to adenocarcinoma. Gastric adenocarcinoma and lymphoma may both present with dyspepsia.

- *History of early satiety*: Seen in linitus plastica and lymphoma and extensive gastric cicatrization due to corrosive intake—all leading to reduced gastric distensibility
- *History of postprandial fullness/heaviness*: Points toward impending gastric outlet obstruction
- *History of vomiting*: Distal gastric lesions cause gastric outlet obstruction, resulting in vomiting, after a few hours of eating. Large in volume, non-bilious and contains partially digested food particles. Bilious vomiting signifies obstruction distal to the second part of the duodenum or toward previous gastric surgery with a Billroth-1/2 reconstruction done likely for peptic ulcer disease
- *History of hematemesis or melena*: Tumoral bleed, generally low volume painless bleed leading to anemia. Whereas GISTs are highly vascular tumors which may cause frank GI bleed.
- *History of postural dizziness, syncope, fatigue, shortness of breath, need for blood transfusion*: Signifies a bleeding tumor and helps to roughly gauge the severity of bleed, which may require some intervention like hemostatic radiotherapy or angioembolization in case the bleed is significant
- *History of loss of weight, loss of appetite*:
  - Beware: LOW happens in benign (corrosive stricture) as well as malignant causes, however LOA happens with malignancy only
- *History of metastatic disease*:
  - Abdominal distension: Due to malignant ascites
  - Dry cough, hemoptysis: Due to pleural effusion and lung metastasis
  - Bony pain, nontraumatic fractures: Due to bony metastasis
  - Unexplained sudden new onset headaches, blackouts, seizures: Due to brain metastasis
- *Treatment history* of having undergone endoscopy, biopsy, administration of chemotherapy, radiotherapy points toward diagnosis of malignant GOO.
- *Past history of any medicines taken for peptic ulcer disease (PUD)? Any surgery?* (Gastrojejunostomy for PUD)
- *History of comorbid illness*: Especially bronchial asthma and COPD which need extensive respiratory optimization before surgery
- *Personal history*: Smoking history—an etiology for malignancy and in anticipation of delayed weaning off ventilator and delayed wound healing
- *Performance history*: As per ECOG (Eastern Cooperative Oncology Group) classification to know if the patient will tolerate surgical stress or at least chemo/radiotherapy.
- *Family history*: Hereditary diffuse gastric cancer due to *CDH-1* gene mutation (it is a germline mutation, autosomal dominant, so progeny have 50% risk of acquiring it). Also history of FAP and Lynch, breast and ovarian tumors (BRCA 1 and 2)

■ EXAMINATION PROFORMA

Same as stated above.

Additional Points for Examination of the Abdomen in Stomach Cancer

On Inspection
- Look for upper abdominal fullness (due to distended stomach)
- Look for any visible lump in the upper abdomen (gastric tumor) and lower abdomen (Krukenberg tumor—metastatic spread to the ovary)
- *If visible, describe*:
  - Size
  - Site
  - Shape
  - Surface
  - Movement with respiration
- *Look for umbilical nodule*: Sister Mary Joseph nodule—points toward metastatic disease similar to Virchow's node (palpable left supra-clavicular node).
- *Look for visible gastric peristalsis*: From left to right in the upper abdomen

On Palpation
- Look for palpable lump
- Gastric tumor in upper abdomen and Krukenberg in lower abdomen in females
- *If present describe*:
  - Site
  - Size
  - Shape
  - Surface
  - Margins
  - Tenderness
  - Consistency
  - Mobility
  - Movement with respiration
- *Plane*:
  - To help differentiate between abdominal wall and intra-abdominal masses, perform the leg raising test (also known as Carnett's test): a parietal mass will become more prominent while the patient raises their legs, while an intra-abdominal mass will become less prominent.
  - To help differentiate between intraperitoneal and retroperitoneal masses, perform the lateral decubitus test: A retroperitoneal mass will not fall ahead, while an intraperitoneal mass will.

On Percussion
Ausculto-percussion test to delineate the outline of greater curvature of the distended stomach.

On Auscultation

Look for succussion splash. Ensure that the ryles tube is not draining, otherwise it will be a false negative test. Ensure that the patient has been fasting for at least 2 hours for liquids and 4 hours for solids, otherwise it will be a false positive test.

For gastric outlet obstruction (GOO), always consider the following differentials:
- *Malignant etiology (if it is a short history spanning a few weeks to months)*:
    - Carcinoma stomach (generally painless). For those presenting with early satiety, postprandial (PP) fullness, first say carcinoma stomach and then if probed, say it could be linitis plastica type adenocarcinoma (adenoCA) or it could be lymphoma (constitutional symptoms may be present).
    - Pancreatic body/tail cancer causing GOO (without jaundice)
    - Chronic pancreatitis (CP) with head mass/head of pancreas (HOP) carcinoma (can present with jaundice, pain and other CP features)
    - Gallbladder cancer (GBC) body/fundus causing GOO (associated with pain and other GBC features, without jaundice)
    - GBC neck (with jaundice)
- *Benign causes (if it is a long history spanning months to years)*:
    - Benign peptic stricture (GERD history)
    - Corrosive stricture (Corrosive history)
- *On imaging, diffuse thickening of stomach wall is seen in*:
    - Linitis plastica
    - Lymphoma
    - Ménétrier's disease [cerebriform gastric folds, protein losing gastropathy, hypoalbuminemia, transforming growth factor alpha (TGF-α) positivity. Cytomegalovirus (CMV) in children and *Helicobacter pylori* in adults can cause this. Treatment is for CMV/*H. pylori*, also cetuximab in some and final resort: gastrectomy]

So now if history is pointing toward malignant causes, say all malignant causes only.

Same with benign.

And if one is more likely than the other, keep the unlikely ones lower down in the list.

After history and examination, always review old records first, starting with upper gastrointestinal endoscopy (UGIE) and biopsy, then USG, chest X-ray (CXR), then baseline investigations (BLI) like hemogram, kidney (KFT) and liver function tests (LFT), then contrast-enhanced computed tomography (CECT), positron emission tomography (PET) CT, and operative records. Then do fresh tests.

So for suspected upper gastrointestinal (UGI) pathology, two sets of investigations, one to arrive/confirm diagnosis, another to complete workup including BLI and other specific tests as need may arise.

Now, for a patient who has presented with bleeding/GOO/is unstable, always resuscitate and ask for BLI first, to know Hb, electrolytes, KFT before going for anything else. A patient presenting with GOO will have hyponatremia, hypokalemia (minor GI, but major renal loss due to excretion of K⁺ in order to save H⁺ ions) with hypochloremic metabolic alkalosis with paradoxical aciduria as kidneys later try to save K⁺ ions by excreting H⁺ ions. So all this needs correction, before going ahead with any staging investigations.

[If platelet count normal, but bleeding time is prolonged, it may be due to platelet functional defects like Glanzmann thrombasthenia or Von Willebrand factor deficiency. Now if all coagulation parameters are ok but still patient is bleeding, he/she may have factor 13 deficiency, which is corrected with fresh frozen plasma (FFP). Thromboelastogram (TEG) when available, helps to diagnose which component of the clotting mechanism is deficient, so that it may be replaced accurately.]

Whereas for a stable patient, always arrive at a diagnosis first, and then proceed to other tests.

So in case of suspected UGI pathology, if patient is stable, then first test will be UGIE with biopsy.

This should be followed by USG abdomen for finding the organ of origin of pathology (if UGIE is normal/inconclusive) and also to rule out obvious metastatic spread) and CXR (to look metastatic spread—cannon ball metastases/effusion).

Then do BLI with relevant tumor markers (as now you know the site of pathology).

Then proceed with CECT for staging, followed by FDG PET CT/DOTATATE PET (as per indications) and then all preoperative fitness evaluation, prehabilitation, preanesthesia checkup (PAC) for risk assessment, multidisciplinary team (MDT) discussion, followed by special preparation few days before and immediate pre-surgical day preparation and actual surgical day preparation and then staging laparoscopy followed by neoadjuvant chemotherapy (NACT)/definitive surgery.

So for a stable patient, to arrive/confirm diagnosis in case of suspected UGI pathology, First ask for UGI with biopsy. Before going for UGIE, put in a Ryles tube, decompress the esophagus/stomach, and in case of GOO, give normal saline (NS) washes.

Siewert Stein type in case of GEJ malignancy:
- *Type I*: Epicenter/of tumor between 1 and 5 cm above GEJ
- *Type II*: Epicenter of tumor between 1 above GEJ and 2 cm below GEJ
- *Type III*: Epicenter of tumor between 2 and 5 cm below GEJ

Try to get biopsy of all lesions before surgery, as treatment depends on it, including chemotherapy/tyrosine kinase inhibitors (TKI)/extent of surgery, etc. So even if imaging looks like adenocarcinoma or gastrointestinal stromal tumor (GIST) or neuroendocrine tumors (NET), get a biopsy done along with immunohistochemistry (IHC). If multiple biopsies are negative, then there is a high likelihood that it may be linitis plastica or lymphoma.

The UGIE report must always mention distance of lesion from upper esophageal sphincter (UES) and from GE Junction, (Siewert is for adenocarcinoma only, so epicenter of lesion should be mentioned), extent of lesion longitudinally and circumferentially and any other associated lesions.

How to increase yield of biopsy:
- Take biopsy from edge of lesion and "well biopsy" aka "biopsy on biopsy" (deeper biopsy)
- 6–8 biopsies in number
- Make use of endoscopic ultrasound (EUS) to take biopsy
- Make use of chromoendoscopy/narrow band imaging (NBI) to take biopsy
    - If biopsy shows poorly differentiated/inconclusive/indeterminate lesion, then immediately ask for IHC, as even lymphoma, GIST and neuroendocrine carcinomas (NEC) can resemble poorly differentiated gastric cancer (GC).
    - If clinically tracheoesophageal fistula (TEF) is suspected, get a barium esophagogram done (use thin barium and not gastrografin, as it can cause pulmonary edema)
- *Next test has to be USG and CXR.*
- Then get BLI done with relevant tumor markers (CEA, CA 19-9, CA 72-4)
- Follow this with CECT IV contrast with neutral oral contrast, neck, chest, abdomen, pelvis. (If it is a nonobstructing esophageal growth, then ask for EUS for T staging as well as N staging and to take EUS FNA/biopsy from lymph node (LN). If tumor is at carinal level/abutting bronchus, ask for bronchoscopy and also, EBUS guided biopsy of peritracheal LN can be done)
- *Indications for doing FDG PET CT (only if patient is not actively bleeding):*
    - For locally advanced (T3/4/N+) proximal tumors (esophagus, GEJ, cardia), if it is not showing any metastases on CECT, then to rule out distant metastases, PET CT is the modality of choice for M staging and changes management in ~25%.
    - Assessing response to NACT (as per NCCN, T2/N+ tumors need NACT. But T2 <3 cm can be taken for upfront surgery) by mRECIST criteria after 2 weeks of NACT [as per MUNICON 1 study: ≥35% reduction in SUV max are labeled responders, and can complete all 12 weeks of NACT. If non-responders, then upfront surgery to be done. In MUNICON 2, they used salvage chemoradiotherapy for non-responders, R0 resection rate did not improve, but major histopathological examination (HPE) response did].
    - Even DW-MRI can be used for response assessment.
    - If PET can be combined with good resolution CECT, then that can be done as a single test, rather than doing CECT followed by PET.
- Follow this up with optimization of comorbidities, nutrition.
- Then staging laparoscopy to be done for all T2/N+ M0, with peritoneal lavage and cytology before starting *NACT and restaging CECT/PET followed by restaging laparoscopy to be done before definitive surgery.*

ESOPHAGUS

Premalignant conditions of esophagus:
- Achalasia cardia [Squamous cell carcinoma (SCC) > adenoCA]
- *Webs*: Patterson Brown Kelly/Plummer Vinson (sideropenic dysphagia with post-cricoid webs and iron deficiency anemia)
- *Peptic etiology*: Barrett's (adenoCA)
- Corrosive stricture
- Tylosis palmaris et plantaris

Cancer

On UGIE: bleeding adenoCA or ulcerated GIST, hemostatic radiotherapy may be given (1,000 Grays).

If on CECT, lesion is proximal to thoracic inlet (formed by T1, 1st pair of ribs and manubrium sterni) or sternal notch (superior part of manubrium), then it is cervical esophagus and treatment is with definitive chemoradiotherapy (CRT).

If lower than that, then do transthoracic esophagectomy (TTE) with extended/total 2 or 3 field. Supraclavicular lymph node (SCLN) is regional for esophageal squamous cell carcinoma (SCC) as prognosis is good with chemotherapy and 3 field surgery, but it is metastatic for GEJ adenocarcinoma because prognosis is poor for it despite chemotherapy and surgery.

Carina is at the level of sternal angle (inferior part of manubrium, at it is junction with sternum), at T4.

If scope could not be passed beyond, and after biopsy and all preoperative imaging patient is operable, then put in a self-expandable metal stent (SEMS) for oral nutrition/put nasojejunal (NJ) tube/do feeding jejunostomy (FJ), then plan for NAC/CRT.

(Before starting any treatment, follow prehabilitation and ERAS—explaining patient the plan, psychological counseling, and then proceeding: Stop smoking/alcohol, oral hygiene, nutrition, incentive spirometry, respiratory muscle training, improving PS by increasing cardiorespiratory fitness by walking, climbing stairs.)

So for SCC, start NACRT as per CROSS protocol [Carboplatin + paclitaxel with 41.4 Gys, 1.8 Gy/day, 23# over 5 weeks, and after reassessment (with PET CT if PET CT was done before, or by CECT) surgery is done 6–8 weeks later. pCR: 49% for SCC and 23% for adenoCA], or

DCF as per NEXT trial by JCOG for esophageal SCC [CF vs. CF-RT vs. DCF, so better overall survival (OS) was seen with DCF].

For adenoCA, latest data from the Neo-AEGIS trial (for esophageal/GEJ adenoCA) [178 CROSS, 184 MAGIC/FLOT (157/27 is split of these 184 patients respectively)]: No evidence that perioperative chemotherapy is unacceptably inferior to multimodal treatment with CROSS. According to HPE regression analysis of the FLOT trial, the pCR rate of the FLOT arm is 16%, which was only 5% in the EOX arm of the Neo-AEGIS trial.

And as per ESOPEC trial, FLOT is better than CROSS.

So for adenoca, FLOT is now the standard of care (SOC).

If NAC/CRT shows near complete/complete metabolic response (seen in 35–40%), in 25–35% it still does not translate to pCR as recurrence is seen within 2 years in these patients. Then salvage esophagectomy can be done, which has higher morbidity, but same OS as seen with esophagectomy done after neoadjuvant treatment.

SANO 1 and 2 are exploring observation versus surgery after 12 weeks NACRT based on Watch and Wait (WW) concept of rectal cancer.

Also, ESOSTRATE, ESOPRESSO and PRIDE trials.

If chemoradiotherapy (CRT) is being given as a palliative intent, then total dose of radiotherapy is 50–60 Grays.

Ideal time for surgery after NACRT: 6–8 weeks, as after 12 weeks there is intense fibrosis.

Before/during/after surgery: Implement ERAS elements and give colon preparation (in readiness for colon conduit).

For surgery: Depending upon the histology and location of the tumor, first decide the field of LN dissection (standard, extended, total 2 or 3 field), and then the site of anastomosis (intrathoracic or cervical) depending on the proximal margin clearance requirement (10 cm for SCC and 5 cm for adenoCA) and surgeon's preference, which will decide which cavity has to be opened—transhiatal esophagectomy (THE) or Ivor Lewis or McKeown.

Total esophagectomy: THE and McKeown

Subtotal: Ivor Lewis

So fields of LN dissection as per ISDE 1994 (which decides which cavity to be opened):
- *Standard 2-field*:
  - Abdominal D2 + paraesophageal LN between subcarinal region, aortopulmonary window and diaphragmatic esophageal hiatus.
- *Extended 2-field*:
  - Standard + Lymph node along right paratracheal gutter along right recurrent laryngeal nerve (RLN) up to brachiocephalic trunk
- *Total 2-field*:
  - Extended + Lymph node along left paratracheal gutter along left RLN
- *3-field*:
  - Total + cervical paraesophageal LN, LN lateral to carotid canal and also SCLN

And there are three approaches to performing the surgery: Open, MIE, and robotic. In open, there are three stages of surgeries (as discussed above: Based on what field of LN dissection is planned and where the anastomosis has to be made—which depends on proximal margin clearance requirement and surgeon's preference):
- Transhiatal esophagectomy
- Transthoracic esophagectomy (TTE) with thoracic anastomosis (Ivor Lewis) aka 2 hole, where dissection is started in the abdomen first
- TTE with cervical anastomosis (McKeown) aka 3 hole, where dissection is started in the chest first

In MIE, there are two types of surgeries:
1. Complete (thoracoscopic and laparoscopic), and hybrid (either thorax or abdomen, done open)
2. Whereas robotic can be completely robotic or partly with MIE/open

Types of conduit:
- If esophageal/GEJ tumor is not involving stomach beyond cardia, then stomach is preferred.
- But if there is extensive involvement of stomach (>5 cm along lesser curvature or involving fundus), then along with esophagectomy, a total gastrectomy needs to be done, and colon must be used as a conduit.
- So in this case, proximal end of colon will be anastomosed to esophagus and distal end to Roux loop of jejunum.

So putting all this together:
- So for distal esophageal SCC, total 2-field LN dissection, TTE with intrathoracic anastomosis (Ivor Lewis) can be done.
- However, if mid/upper thoracic SCC, total 2-/3-field LN dissection if RLN sentinel node (SN) + [as there is a higher chance of spread to cervical lymph node (LNs)], TTE with cervical anastomosis (McKeown) should be done (proximal margin clearance of at least 10 cm required for esophageal SCC).
- For distal esophageal adenoCA and Siewert 1 and 2, extended/total 2-field, TTE with intrathoracic anastomosis can be done.
- Even for more proximal esophageal adenoCA, a maximum of total 2-field should be done, as 3-field does not add to OS for adenoCA.
- Remember that for any TTE, thoracic or cervical anastomosis can be done depending upon proximal margin clearance (at least 10 cm for SCC and 5 cm for adenoCA) and comfort of surgeon.
- Transhiatal esophagectomy should be done for lower esophageal/GEJ adenoca only if 5 cm proximal margin and at least lower paraesophageal LN clearance (ideally up to subcarinal region and aortopulmonary window, with the help of retractors and telescopes, under vision, as described by Orringer) can be achieved. For Siewert 3, transhiatal extended D2 gastrectomy is an oncologically adequate procedure. Also, for benign esophageal pathology, THE is a valid option.
- Apart from these indications, THE is only done to reduce pulmonary morbidity in high risk patients, who would have otherwise warranted a TTE.
- Just remember that latest Japanese GC guidelines permit THE with lower mediastinal LN clearance for junctional CA invading up to 4 cm into esophagus. For >4 cm invasion, even they advise TTE with mid and upper mediastinal LN clearance.

TTE with thoracic anastomosis (Ivor Lewis), problems are:
- Proximal margin clearance lesser than with total esophagectomy
- Higher morbidity of leak
- Troublesome esophagogastric reflux

TTE with cervical anastomosis (McKeown), problems are:
- Higher leak rate

CHAPTER 2.1: Upper Gastrointestinal—Esophagus and Stomach Cases

- Lesser pulmonary morbidity (but 60% can still have serious complications like mediastinitis and pulmonary abscess due to infection tracking down the fascial spaces)

THE (obviously with cervical anastomosis), problems are:
- Mediastinal LN clearance inadequate
- Higher chance of intrathoracic bleeding, tracheal injury, RLN injury in neck, and conduit ischemia, necrosis, stricture due to long distance.

HIVEX trial: Open TTE versus THE, so TTE better for esophageal SCC while THE can be done for GEJ adenoca. But in a subgroup analysis of Siewert type 1 cancer, better long term OS with TTE (64% vs. 23%) in those with a limited number of positive LN, from 1–8.

TIME: Minimally invasive esophagectomy (MIE) versus open TTE, so MIE better short term outcomes and oncologically same.

Minimally invasive surgery avoids thoracotomy anyway, so then MIE (thoracoscopic and laparoscopic) becomes obvious procedure of choice.

ICAN trial: Cervical versus thoracic anastomosis after MIE. So cervical has better margin clearance, more leak, less morbidity after leak. Thoracic has more positive margins, less leak but higher morbidity after leak

MIRO: Hybrid versus open TTE, so even hybrid has reduced risk of pulmonary morbidity.

ROBOT: Robotic (RAMIE) versus open TTE, so robotic has better short-term outcomes.
- For cT4b lesions, RAMIE or open TTE is preferred over MIE to be careful with membranous trachea.

Akiyama et al. before the advent of NACRT:
- 3-field LN dissection better OS.

Rizk et al. WECC database (retrospective) in patients without NACRT:
- Number of LN to be removed are at least 10, 20 and 30 for T1, T2 and T3/4 respectively.
- Helps in better staging and even better OS.

Recent meta-analysis, Swedish, Netherlands studies post-NACRT:
- 3-field improves OS without increasing morbidity, mortality.

If upfront surgery has been done due to bleeding/obstruction without knowing diagnosis, then if HPE is SCC, and even if nodes are uninvolved, best to get a PET done now, and discuss with oncologist for chemoradiotherapy as LN dissection may not be adequate and also because SCC involves distant nodes/has skip nodal metastases as well.

Achalasia

Halitosis seen due to stagnant food, so it is seen in chronic esophageal obstructive pathologies like benign stricture, achalasia and zenkers, as in these conditions, esophagus becomes dilated and roomy to accomodate food.

This is generally not seen with cancer.

DDs are:
- Schatzki ring (always seen with hiatus hernia)
- Other lower esophageal webs/rings
- Peptic stricture
- Corrosive stricture
- Lower esophageal/GEJ/proximal stomach carcinoma.

Sequence of investigations in achalasia: Chest X-ray, timed barium esophagogram (TBE), UGIE and high-resolution manometry (HRM).

What to look for in CXR of achalasia:
- Bilateral lung fields for consolidation, effusion
- Mediastinal widening
- Air fluid level in esophagus
- Absence of fundic air shadow

Before doing barium esophagogram (BE)/UGIE, first put a Ryles tube, decompress, only then go ahead.

So finding on BE: All above + tortuosity of esophagus, axis deviation (depends on alpha angle), dilatation <3.5, 3.5–6, >6 cm.

So >6 cm dilatation is mega esophagus, and if tortuosity and axis deviation also present, then it is termed as sigmoid esophagus. Bird beak appearance and Hurst phenomenon are seen on barium esophagogram.

TBE: 100–250 mL of 45% barium sulphate ingested as quickly as possible, then films taken at 1, 2, and 5 minutes and height and width of column recorded in each film.
- Shows width, morphology, axis deviation of esophagus
- Denotes volume of barium emptied at timed intervals.
- Helps to confirm diagnosis and to assess treatment response objectively.

Before UGIE also, always decompress esophagus with Ryles tube, else patient may aspirate. So UGIE done to:
- See dilatation, residual food and to evaluate mucosa for stasis esophagitis, any ulcers, any malignant change due to long standing achalasia (secondary to achalasia, adenoCA can develop at site of air fluid level while SCC at mid/lower site)
- Evaluate for viral/fungal disease
- Rule out carcinoma causing pseudoachalasia

High-resolution manometry shows esophageal pressure topography map:
- Helps to classify motility disorders as per Chicago 4 **(Flowchart 1)**
- Helps to decide treatment: So for type 3 achalasia, distal esophageal spasm (DES) and hypercontractile esophagus, per-oral endoscopic myotomy (POEM) is the treatment of choice, followed by modified laparoscopic Heller's myotomy (LHM), but more acid reflux and esophagitis seen after POEM and long-term outcomes are pending. Whereas for type 1 and 2 achalasia, pneumatic dilatation (PD) and LHM have almost equivalent outcomes, but PD requires multiple sessions and there is a definite risk of perforation. Also, POEM can be used as well.
- Helps to assess treatment response. So, if lower esophageal sphincter (LES) pressure is <10 mm Hg after PD or LHM, then it is successful intervention.

CHAPTER 2.1: Upper Gastrointestinal—Esophagus and Stomach Cases

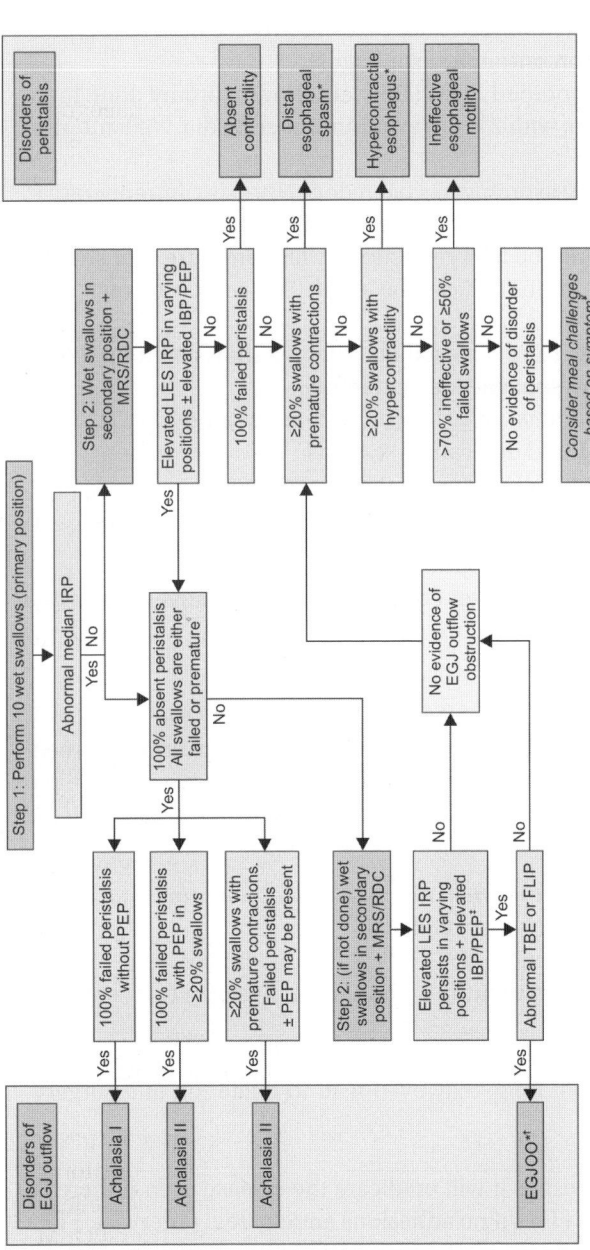

FLOWCHART 1: Chicago 4 Classification.[1]

* Denote manometric patterns of unclear clinical relevance. A clinically relevant conclusive diagnosis requires additional information which may include clinically relevant symptoms and/or supportive testing (as detailed in the document).

† Patients with EGJ obstruction and presence of peristaltic swallows would fulfill strict criteria for EGJOO and may have features suggestive of achalasia or other patterns of peristalsis defined by criteria for disorders of peristalsis: EGJOO with spastic features, EGJOO with hypercontractile esophagus, EGJOO with ineffective motility, or EGJOO with no evidence of disordered peristalsis.

‡ RDC, solid test swallows, and/or pharmacologic provocation with amyl nitrite or cholecystokinin (if available) can be instituted here to assess for obstruction.

◊ Patients previously defined absent contractility based on 10 swallows in the primary position may have achalasia if the IRP is elevated in the alternate position, with the RDC, and/or with MRS. These cases should be considered inconclusive for type I or II achalasia as appropriate and evaluated further with TBE/FLIP.

¥ If no evidence of a disorder of peristalsis or EGJ outflow in a patient with high probability of a missed EGJOO, a solid test meal can be added to rule out an obstructive pattern; if abnormal then the possibility of a mechanical obstruction should be readdressed. In a patient with regurgitation or belching, post-prandial high-resolution impedance monitoring can be used to assess for rumination/belching disorder.

(IRP: integrated relaxation pressure; MRS: multiple rapid swallow; RDC: rapid drink challenge; LES: lower esophageal sphincter; IBP: intrabolus pressurization; PEP: panesophageal pressurization; EGJ: esophagogastric junction; EGJOO: EGJ outflow obstruction; TBE: timed barium esophagram; FLIP: functional lumen imaging probe)

PD: Graded dilatation done with Rigiflex balloon—
- 3, 3.5, 4 cm over 1–2 minutes. When streak of blood is seen, it means that dilatation has been completed.
  - Advantages of POEM over LHM: Incisionless, no intra-abdominal adhesions, and longer myotomy (16 cm vs. 8 cm), hence better for type 3 achalasia, DES and hypercontractile esophagus.
  - What to remember in modified LHM: Only anterior myotomy done for a maximum length of 8 cm, with 2–3 cm extending over cardia, with anterior Dor fundoplication.
  - How to ensure adequate myotomy has been done: By using intraoperative manometry, to see reduction in pressure after myotomy (aka calibrated myotomy, so there should be 50% reduction in LES pressure or it should be <10 mm Hg), also EndoFLIP can be used (to see compliance and distensibility)
  - Advantages of Toupet over Dor: Latest meta-analysis shows both similar in terms of postoperative dysphagia and acid reflux.
  - Type of diet in postoperative of LHM (do a contrast study POD1, start liquids, and POD2 semisolid diet can be started)
  - Follow-up 3 monthly with Eckardt score, TBE, manometry

So procedure is a success if:
- Eckardt score <3 or decrease by ≥3 points
- On TBE if >50% is emptied at 5 minutes compared to preoperative
- On manometry, if LES pressure <10 mm

Esophageal Stricture

If benign esophageal smooth esophageal stricture/indeterminate stricture seen on BE, and if endoscopic/EUS guided biopsy and CECT findings are also benign then PET CT should be done. Submucosal fibrosis causing stricture can be seen with lymphoma/TB too.

So after all this if it is a benign stricture, then management options are:
- Endoscopic dilatation (balloon/savary Gillard)
- Endoscopic steroid/botox injection
- If failure of endoscopic management (>5 sessions in 3 weeks) then counsel for surgery
- If emaciated, then before surgery put a fully covered SEMS (FC-SEMS), build up nutrition and if placed for long, may even lead to dilatation and surgery may not be needed.
- *Surgical options are*:
  - Esophagectomy is the best as it will eradicate the disease even if there is any focus of malignancy (THE if no adhesions anticipated, otherwise TTE. If expertise for MIE is there, then MIE preferred)
  - Esophageal bypass with colonic/jejunal conduit only if 100% sure that it is benign or when esophagectomy is going to be very morbid (dense periesophageal adhesions)

■ STOMACH

If patient presents with GOO and it is adenocarcinoma, and if CECT shows no metastases, then do staging laparoscopy to stage. If no metastases and peritoneal cytology negative, then put nasojejunal tube (NJT) for feeding access and consider perioperative chemotherapy for cT2/N+ disease.

If metastases+, then can do palliative resection (for resectable bleeding or resectable GOO) or bypass (if unresectable tumor) if patient can tolerate, or just do feeding jejunostomy (FJ) and start palliative chemotherapy.

If it is lymphoma with GOO, then put or do FJ, avoid resection as far as possible and then start chemo/radiotherapy as soon as possible, as resection will delay chemo/radiotherapy, which is the actual treatment.

Gastric Cancer

Few essential definitions and management principles of gastric cancer (GC) as per Japanese GC treatment guidelines.[2]

Types and Definitions of Gastric Surgery

Standard gastrectomy and non-standard gastrectomy in surgery with curative intent.

Standard Gastrectomy

Principal surgical procedure performed with curative intent. Involves resection of at least two-thirds of the stomach with a D2 lymph node dissection.

Non-standard Gastrectomy

Extent of gastric resection and/or lymphadenectomy is determined depending on tumor stage. It includes modified surgery and extended surgery.

Modified Surgery

The extent of gastric resection and/or lymphadenectomy is reduced (D1, D1+, etc.), compared to standard surgery.

Extended Surgery

- Gastrectomy with combined resection of adjacent involved organs.
- Gastrectomy with extended lymphadenectomy exceeding D2.

Non-curative Surgery

Palliative Surgery

- Palliative gastrectomy or gastrojejunostomy done for bleeding or obstruction, in a patient with advanced/metastatic gastric cancer.
- Reported to result in maintaining quality of life, improvement of oral intake and a good prognosis

Margins

A proximal margin of at least 3 cm is recommended for T2 or deeper tumors with an expansive growth pattern (types 1 and 2) and 5 cm for those with an infiltrative growth pattern (types 3 and 4).

Selection of Gastrectomy

The standard surgical procedure for clinically node-positive (cN+) or T2–T4a tumors is either total or distal gastrectomy.

Even in a case that a satisfactory proximal resection margin can be obtained, pancreatic invasion by tumor requiring pancreaticosplenectomy necessitates total gastrectomy regardless of the tumor location. Total gastrectomy with splenectomy should be considered for tumors that are located along the greater curvature.

For cT1N0 tumors, the following types of gastric resection can be considered according to tumor location.

- *Pylorus-preserving gastrectomy (PPG)*: For tumors in the middle portion of the stomach with the distal tumor border at least 4 cm proximal from the pylorus.
- *Proximal gastrectomy*: For proximal tumors where more than half of the distal stomach can be preserved.

Lymph Node Dissection

Total Gastrectomy

- *D0*: Lymphadenectomy less than D1
- *D1*: Nos. 1–7
- *D1+*: D1 + Nos. 8a, 9, 11p
- *D2*: D1 + Nos. 8a, 9, 11p, 11d, 12a

For tumors invading the esophagus, resection of Nos. 19, 20, and 110* should be added to D2

Distal Gastrectomy

- *D0*: Lymphadenectomy less than D1
- *D1*: Nos. 1, 3, 4sb, 4d, 5, 6, 7
- *D1+*: D1 + Nos. 8a, 9
- *D2*: D1 + Nos. 8a, 9, 11p, 12a

Proximal Gastrectomy

- *D0*: Lymphadenectomy less than D1
- *D1*: Nos. 1, 2, 3a, 4sa, 4sb, 7
- *D1+*: D1 + Nos. 8a, 9, 11p
- *D2*: D1 + Nos. 8a, 9, 11p, 11d

For tumors invading the esophagus, Nos. 19, 20, and 110* should additionally be dissected in D2

---

*No. 110 lymph nodes (lower thoracic para-esophageal nodes) in gastric cancer invading the esophagus are those attached to the lower part of the esophagus that is removed to obtain a sufficient resection margin.

Indications for Lymph Node Dissection

D2 lymphadenectomy is indicated for cN + or ≥ cT2 tumors and a D1 or D1+ for cT1N0 tumors. Since pre- and intraoperative diagnoses regarding the depth of tumor invasion and nodal involvement remain unreliable, D2 lymphadenectomy should be performed whenever the possibility of nodal involvement cannot be dismissed.

D1 Lymphadenectomy

For cT1a tumors that do not meet the criteria for EMR/ESD, and for cT1bN0 tumors that are histologically of differentiated type and 1.5 cm or smaller in diameter.

D1 + Lymphadenectomy

For cT1N0 tumors other than the above.

D2 Lymphadenectomy

For potentially curable cT2-T4 tumors, as well as cT1N+tumors. The spleen should be preserved in total gastrectomy for advanced cancer of the proximal stomach provided the tumor does not involve the greater curvature.

D2 + Lymphadenectomy

Gastrectomy with extended lymphadenectomy beyond D2 is classified as a non-standard gastrectomy, and could be considered for the following cases, although hard evidence is lacking, on the condition that it can be conducted safely.
- Dissection of No. 10 (splenic hilar lymph nodes) with or without splenectomy for cancer of the proximal stomach invading the greater curvature (D2 + No. 10).
- Dissection of No. 14v (superior mesenteric venous lymph node) for cancer of the distal stomach with metastasis to the No. 6 lymph nodes (D2 + No. 14v).
- Dissection of No. 13 (posterior pancreas head lymph node) for cancer invading the duodenum (D2 + No. 13). Metastases to the No. 13 nodes, which are not included in the regional lymph nodes for gastric cancer, should usually be classified as M1. However, since the No. 13 nodes are among the regional lymph nodes for cancer of the duodenum according to the TNM classification and the Japanese Classification of Gastric Carcinoma 15th edition, these should be regarded as regional lymph nodes once gastric cancer invades the duodenum.
- Dissection of No. 16 (abdominal aortic lymph node) after neoadjuvant chemotherapy for cancer with extensive lymph node involvement (D2 + No. 16)

Management of Junctional Cancer

For junctional CA (epicentre ≤2 cm of GEJ)/proximal stomach cancer invading esophagus, as per Nishi classification, latest Japanese GC guidelines (6e) are:
- *Up to 4 cm esophageal invasion*: THE with clearance of lower mediastinal paraesophageal LN (19, 20, 110) can be done.

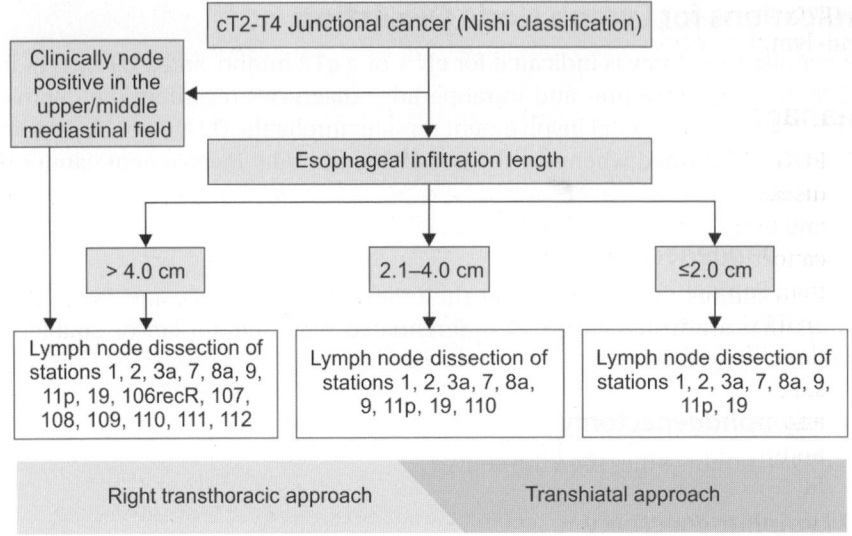

FLOWCHART 2: Nishi classification.[2]

- *>4 cm*: TTE with middle and upper mediastinal LN clearance needs to be done **(Flowchart 2)**.

Omentectomy

For T1/T2 tumors, the omentum more than 3 cm away from the gastroepiploic artery may be preserved. Removal of the greater omentum is usually integrated in the standard gastrectomy for T3 or deeper tumors. A clinical trial confrming the non-inferiority of omentum preservation to omentectomy for T3 or deeper tumors (JCOG1711) is underway.

Bursectomy

The survival beneft of this procedure has been denied by a large-scale, randomized trial (JCOG1001), not only for all enrolled patients, but also for subsets with T4a tumors and tumors located in the posterior wall.

Stump Carcinoma DDs

- Stomal stenosis leading to obstruction
- Jejunogastric intussusception
- Retrocolic GJ done in a distended stomach away from pylorus may not drain properly after many years as stomach shrinks and GJ moves up

Staging for stump carcinoma should include USG abdomen, CXR, then CECT, then even FDG PET CT (as it mostly presents as an advanced disease) and staging lap, followed by perioperative chemotherapy (FLOT is preferred in poorly differentiated and has better pCR and OS than ECF, but increased toxicity), surgery being completion D2 gastrectomy with resection of jejunal limbs along with lymph nodes of the involved mesentery.

Management of Oligometastatic GC

- FDG PET CT is done before staging laparoscopy only for locally advanced disease, whereas all patients with T2/N+ disease undergo staging laparoscopy and peritoneal wash cytology (PC), (IHC wherein antibodies are used against cancer cells/RT-PCR wherein the cancer cell genes are identified, are better than Pap stain based cytology).
- So if PC+, and no macroscopic disease (no nodules) and no other metastases, then this is defined as CY1 by the Japanese GC guidelines and is considered stage 4, M1 disease. Traditionally this has been considered inoperable, and patients were sent for palliative chemo, but in recent years, treatment approaches have developed.
- So two approaches:
  i. Conversion chemotherapy (try to downstage with chemo, make it PC negative) as per FLOT3 trial:
     - So give 4 cycles (4#) of neoadjuvant chemotherapy (NACT) (FLOT), then do restaging laparoscopy with wash. If restaging now shows PC−, then proceed with D2 gastrectomy and complete the perioperative chemotherapy (remaining 4# FLOT).
     - But if restaging still shows PC+, or if macroscopic disease/other metastases develop, then it is considered progressive disease (PD) and palliative chemo is still the standard of care.
  ii. Upfront surgery followed by adjuvant chemotherapy:
     - So latest Japanese GC guidelines (6e) for CY1, permit D2 gastrectomy followed by S1 adjuvant chemotherapy with 5 year survival of 25%.

  Remember that even for solitary liver metastases confined to liver or for bulky 16a2/b1 [ParaAortic Lymph Node (PALN+)], Japanese GC guidelines permit NACT followed by D2 gastrectomy and resection of the liver metastases/PALN.
- So now if staging laparoscopy initially had shown peritoneal nodules or liver metastases, or if it is a PD even after NACT (i.e., still PC+, or development of peritoneal nodules or organ metastases), then palliative chemo is still the standard of care. However, recent reports from Europe, have shown that for highly select individuals [good PS, chemotherapy responsive, and oligometastatic disease: <5 metastases in liver or PALN+ or limited macroscopic peritoneal disease with peritoneal carcinomatosis index (PCI) ≤6 or PC+], perioperative chemotherapy (4# FLOT before and after surgery as per FLOT3 protocol) along with D2 gastrectomy, CRS and HIPEC have a better survival than only palliative chemotherapy.

Studies for curative surgery for oligometastatic/peritoneal disease:
- REGATTA trial enrolled GC patients with a single non-curable factor (liver, PALN or peritoneum) to chemo alone or gastrectomy only followed by chemo. In contrast to the FLOT3 results, this trial failed to show improvements in

survival for surgically treated patients and even showed a trend toward inferiority in the surgery group (median OS was 16.6 months in patients without vs. 14.3 months in patients with gastrectomy). However, the design of the study is highly debatable, as gastrectomy was restricted to D1 without resection of any metastases.
- Whereas FLOT3 showed OS 31 months for NACT of 4# FLOT followed by curative resection of primary with metastases followed by adjuvant chemo of 4# FLOT versus 16 months for 8# FLOT with non-curative resection.
- FLOT3 protocol was carried forward in FLOT4 study (FLOT vs. ECF) for resectable GC, and FLOT4 became the new standard for perioperative chemotherapy.
- FLOT5/Renaissance and SURGIGAST is ongoing study for surgery in oligometastatic GEJ/gastric adenoCA.
- *CONVO GC*: Better OS with NACT and surgery for metastases
- *CYTO CHIP study for peritoneal metastases positive GC*: CRS–HIPEC improves OS compared with CRS alone.
- *GASTRIPEC study for peritoneal metastases positive GC*: CRS + HIPEC versus CRS alone. So HIPEC did not add to OS, but improved progression free survival (PFS) and other metastatic free survival. Problem with study was that almost 50% had PCI > 7 with ascites which are poor prognostic factors. But subgroup analysis still showed, that for patients undergoing complete cytoreduction, there was definite increase in OS in CRS + HIPEC group compared with CRS alone.

GI Lymphoma

Staging systems (**Table 1 and Box 1**).

TABLE 1: Lugano and Paris staging systems for gastrointestinal lymphomas[3,4]

Lugano staging system		Paris staging system	Tumor extension
Stage I	Tumor confined to the GI tract (single primary site or multiple, noncontiguous lesions)	• T1m N0 M0 • T1sm N0 M0 • T2 N0 M0 • T3 N0 M0	• Mucosa • Submucosa • Muscularis propria • Serosa
Stage II	Tumor extending into abdomen	—	—
II₁	Local nodal involvement	T1–3 N1 M0	Perigastric lymph nodes
II₂	Distant nodal involvement	T1–3 N2 M0	More distant regional nodes

Continued

Continued

Lugano staging system		Paris staging system	Tumor extension
Stage IIE	Penetration of serosa to involve adjacent organs or tissues	T4 N0–2 M0	Invasion of adjacent structures with or without abdominal lymph nodes
Stage IV	Disseminated extranodal involvement or concomitant supradiaphragmatic nodal involvement	• T1–4 N3 M0 • T1–4 N0–3 M1 • T1–4 N0–3 M2	• Extra-abdominal lymph nodes and/or additional distant GI sites or non-GI sites
		• T1–4 N0–3 M0–2 deeper biopsy	• Bone marrow not assessed
		• T1–4 N0–3 M0–2 B0	• Bone marrow not involved
		• T1–4 N0–3 M2 B1	• Bone marrow involvement

Box 1: The international prognostic index[5]

One point is assigned for each of the following risk factors:
- Age greater than 60 years
- Stage III or IV disease
- Elevated serum LDH
- ECOG/Zubrod performance status of 2, 3, or 4
- More than 1 extranodal site

The sum of the points allotted correlates with the following risk groups:
- Low risk (0–1 points): 5-year survival of 73%
- Low-intermediate risk (2 points): 5-year survival of 51%
- High-intermediate risk (3 points): 5-year survival of 43%
- High risk (4–5 points): 5-year survival of 26%

Treatment of Gastric Lymphomas

Chemoradiotherapy is the primary modality of treatment.

For DLBCL, Mantle cell lymphoma, follicular cell lymphoma:
RCHOP +/− Radiotherapy
R: Rituximab (anti-CD-20 mAb)
C: Cyclophosphamide
H: Doxorubicin
O: Vincristine (oncovin)
P: Prednisolone

For Burkitt lymphoma:
CHOM (M-Methotrexate)

For Maltoma:
- *H. pylori with t(11,18)*: H. pylori treatment + ISRT/rituximab
- *H. pylori without translocation*: Just H. pylori treatment
- *H. pylori negative*: Just ISRT
- *Stage 4 MALTOMA*: RCHOP/4 cycles of rituximab +/- Radiotherapy

Surgery only for emergency indications like obstruction, perforation, bleeding and when preoperative diagnosis is not possible.

Similarly, for other GI lymphomas, rituximab/ISRT is the treatment of choice and surgery is done only for emergency indications as listed above.

Also for stage 4 nongastric MALTOMA, RCHOP is the treatment of choice.

Gastrointestinal Stromal Tumor (GIST)

- *Irrespective of imaging findings, always get a biopsy with IHC done.*
- So anyway, in a probable GIST, preoperative biopsy with IHC and mutational analysis helps to plan type of neoadjuvant (NA) treatment with tyrosine kinase inhibitors (TKI) (required in GIST if size ≥10 cm or for organ preservation, to avoid morbidity a major resection, like when near GEJ/rectal GISTs near dentate line) and also to know whether LN dissection is required (SDH deficient and pediatric GISTS have LN involvement). Also, risk stratification based on mitotic index, size, and site must be done for prognosticating.
- CECT is done for staging disease.
- On resected specimen always get IHC done. Risk stratification to be done as per AFIP or modified Joensuu (NIH) criteria, for deciding need for adjuvant treatment. (High-risk GISTs: Mitotic index >10/50 HPF or 5 mm^2, size >10 cm, or mitotic index and size both >5, nongastric site and tumor rupture, need adjuvant imatinib 400 mg/day at least for 3 years, as per ACOSOG and PERSIST trials).
- R1 resection has equal OS like R0, so no need for re-resection and some groups say that even in such a case if it is a low-risk GIST, then imatinib can be avoided.
- Always get mutational analysis, as exon 11 (mostly found in gastric GISTs) responds well to imatinib 400 mg/day, but mutation in exon 9 (remember as N for nine, not good and iNtestiNal) needs double dose imatinib at 800 mg/day and PDGFRA 842V mutation does not respond to imatinib, but responds to avapritinib (BLU-285). Also if KIT, PDGFRA, BRAF wild type, then test for SDH deficiency (points to syndromic GISTs seen with Carney triad, Carney Stratakis and pediatric GISTs) and for NF1, both of which do not respond to imatinib.
- If imatinib resistant, start sunitinib at 37.5 mg/day continuous treatment or regorafinib 160 mg daily (3 weeks on, 1 week off) as third line or even pazopanib can be given. Even if resistant, keep continuing treatment, and changing back to imatinib even though resistant, does help as it slows progression. But stopping imatinib leads to quick recurrence, so never stop tyrosine kinase inhibitors.

- *Side effects of all three tyrosine kinase inhibitors*: Nausea, vomiting, diarrhea, fatigue, all three cytopenias, deranged LFTs, hypothyroidism. Sunitinib also causes hand foot mouth syndrome.
- For metastatic GIST, imatinib is 1st line, response assessed with FDG PET CT by modified Choi criteria (tumor size and density). Increased density/nodule in mass = progression. No response, then double the dose. If still no response, then change to 2nd/3rd line, and if still no response, then shift back to imatinib and continue life-long.
- Watch and Wait policy for GIST <2 cm, keep on follow-up with UGIE and EUS.

Neuroendocrine Neoplasm (NEN)

- Biopsy is done to know differentiation (well or poorly) and grade (based on mitotic rate and Ki-67) as per latest WHO classification.
- Well-differentiated neuroendocrine neoplasms (NENs) are called neuroendocrine tumors (NETs), and can be Grades—G1, G2, G3 while poorly differentiated neuroendocrine neoplasm are called neuroendocrine carcinomas (NECs), are always G3, and have a poor prognosis **(Tables 2 and 3)**.

Management of Localized Gastric NETs

- *Type 1*: Endoscopic removal
- *Type 2*: Surgical removal of gastrinoma with endoscopic removal of gastric lesions
- *Type 3*: D2 Gastrectomy to be done
- *Type 4*: Multiple small lesions with hypertrophy and hyperplasia of parietal cells with vacuolated cytoplasm—structural abnormality prevents the HCL from being secreted, leading to achlorhydria, hypergastrinemia and hyperplasia of neuroendocrine cells
- D2 Gastrectomy to be done

TABLE 2: WHO 2019 classification of GEP NEN[6]

Terminology	Differentiation	Grade	Mitotic rate[a]	Ki-67 index[b]
NET, G1	Well-differentiated	Low	<2	<3%
NET, G2		Intermediate	2–20	3–20%
NET, G3		High	>20	>20%
SCNEC	Poorly differentiated	High	>20	>20%
LCNEC			>20	>20%
MiNEN	Well or poorly differentiated	Variable	Variable	Variable

[a] Mitotic rate, number of mitoses per 2 mm².
[b] Ki-67 index, counting ≥500 cells in the regions of highest labeling (hot-spots) which are identified at scanning magnification.

(LCNEC: large cell neuroendocrine carcinoma; MiNEN: mixed neuroendocrine non-neuroendocrine neoplasm; NEC: neuroendocrine carcinoma; NENs: neuroendocrine neoplasms; NET: neuroendocrine tumor; SCNEC: small cell neuroendocrine carcinoma)

TABLE 3: GASTRIC neuroendocrine neoplasm types[7]

	Gastric neuroendocrine tumors (NETs)/carcinoids		
	Type 1	Type 2	Type 3
Relative frequency	70–80%	5–6%	14–25%
Features	Mostly small (<1–2 cm) and multiple	Mostly small (<1–2 cm) and multiple	Solitary, often >2 cm
Associated conditions	CAG	MEN1/ZES[a]	No
Histology	Well-differentiated G1[b]	Well-differentiated G1[b]	Well/moderate-differentiated G2
Serum gastrin	(Very) high	(Very) high	Normal
Gastric pH	Anacidic	Hyperacidic	Normal
Metastases	<10%	10–30%	50–100%
Tumor-related death	No	<10%	25–30%

[a] Zollinger–Ellison syndrome.
[b] Grade 1.
Note: Clinicopathological characteristics of gastric neuroendocrine neoplasms.

NECs, however, have poor prognosis overall—for localized lesions surgery may have some benefit, however for metastatic NEC, platinum based chemotherapy is the only treatment.

Management of Metastatic Gastric NETs

So surgery (for primary as well as for resectable metastases), everolimus, sunitinib, somatostatin analogs, peptide receptor radionuclide therapy (PRRT) are effective treatment options for Grade 1 and 2 NETs, whereas surgery (for primary as well as for resectable metastases) and Capecitabine-Temozolomide (CapTem) chemotherapy are effective for G3 NET. Platinum based chemotherapy alone (carboplatin/etoposide) is the treatment for metastatic G3 NEC **(Fig. 1 and Table 4)**.

Debulking for G1/G2 and even some G3 NETs should be done if >90% or even >70% liver disease (latest reports) can be removed and if primary is resectable (however, increase in OS is seen with debulking with liver metastatic burden even if primary is unresectable as liver metastases decide prognosis always, and not the primary).

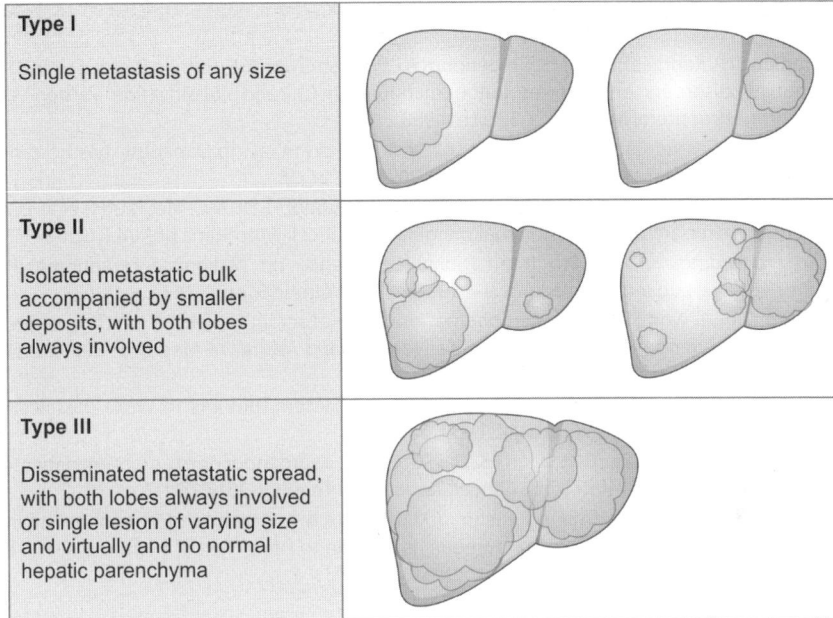

Type I	Single metastasis of any size
Type II	Isolated metastatic bulk accompanied by smaller deposits, with both lobes always involved
Type III	Disseminated metastatic spread, with both lobes always involved or single lesion of varying size and virtually and no normal hepatic parenchyma

FIG. 1: Frilling classification of neuroendocrine liver metastasis (NELM).[8]

TABLE 4: Management of NELM as per Frilling classification

Patterns of NEN-LM (neuroendocrine neoplasm liver metastases)

Type	Description
I	• "Restricted metastases", metastases confined to one liver lobe or limited to two adjacent segments • *Prevalence*: 20–25% • *Resectability*: Metastases are clearly resectable with a standard anatomical resection
II	• "Dominant lesion with bilobar metastases", in which there is one dominant lesion but with smaller satellites contralaterally • *Prevalence*: 10–15% • *Resectability*: Metastases may be potentially resectable and can be approached surgically with a combination of ablative therapy on the contralateral lobe
III	• "Diffuse, multifocal liver metastases" • *Prevalence*: 60–70% of the cases • *Resectability*: Surgery is not an option as clearly unresectable. Liver transplant may be considered for these tumors

REFERENCES

1. Yadlapati R, Kahrilas PJ, Fox MR, Bredenoord AJ, Prakash Gyawali C, Roman S, et al. Esophageal motility disorders on high-resolution manometry: Chicago classification version 4.0©. Neurogastroenterol Motil. 2021;33(1):e14058.
2. Japanese Gastric Cancer Association jgca@ koto. kpu-m. ac. jp. Japanese gastric cancer treatment guidelines 2021. Gastric Cancer. 2023;26(1):1-25.
3. Ruskone-Fourmestraux A, Fischbach W, Aleman BMP, Boot H, Du MQ, Megraud F, et al. EGILS consensus report. Gastric extranodal marginal zone B-cell lymphoma of MALT. Gut 2011.
4. In Proceedings of the 5th International Conference on Malignant Lymphoma, Part Proceedings, Lugano, Switzerland, 9–12 June 1994; Volume 5, pp. 1-163.
5. International Non-Hodgkin's Lymphoma Prognostic Factors Project. A predictive model for aggressive non-Hodgkin's lymphoma. New England Journal of Medicine. 1993;329(14): 987-94.
6. Klimstra DS, Kloppel G, La Rosa S, Rindi G. Digestive System Tumours. In: WHO Classification of Tumours. 5th edition. Vol 1. IARC, Lyon, 2019.
7. Kwon DH, Nakakura EK, Bergsland EK, Dai SC. Gastric neuroendocrine tumors: management and challenges. Gastrointestinal Cancer: Targets and Therapy. 2017;7:31-7.
8. Frilling A, Li J, Malamutmann E, Schmid KW, Bockisch A, Broelsch CE. Treatment of liver metastases from neuroendocrine tumours in relation to the extent of hepatic disease. Br J Surg. 2009;96(2):175-84.

2.2 CHAPTER

Upper Gastrointestinal— Corrosive Injury

Professor Ananthakrishnan and Professor Vikram Kate have worked extensively on corrosive injuries. The following section is guided by their principles of managing this calamity.

■ DYSPHAGIA DUE TO CORROSIVE INJURY

History

1. *History of corrosive consumption (alleged), nature of corrosive consumed, i.e., acidic or alkaline, intent of consumption, whether suicidal or accidental, and whether patient was under abuse of any substance at that point of time*:
   - Acid ingestion is seen more often in India.
     – Toilet cleaners like harpic are acids.
     – Acids are pungent, hence consumed in less amount, and cause coagulative necrosis [except hydrofluoric (HF) acid causing liquefactive necrosis] and eschar formation, and thus are not expected to cause transmural esophageal injury, but more of gastric injury due to stasis resulting from reflux pylorospasm. However it's been seen that they cause extensive injury to esophagus as well.
     – Bathroom floor and Vessel cleaners are alkalis.
     – Alkalis are odorless, tasteless, hence consumed in more amount, and cause liquefactive necrosis and are viscous, so stick to esophageal mucosa, thus causing extensive esophageal injury as compared to gastric injury.
   - Suicidal consumption: Hesitancy leads to severe injury to oral cavity, oropharynx, pharyngoesophageal junction, upper esophagus and airways.
   - Accidental consumption or consumption under influence of drugs/ alcohol: Large volume rapid consumption, causes more of distal esophageal, stomach, rarely duodenal injury.
   - Day and time of consumption: To know the total duration of the disease.
2. *Symptoms soon afterward to know the severity of the injury*: Asymptomatic/ mild throat pain points toward milder injury. Odynophagia, dysphagia,

drooling of saliva, hematemesis, chest pain, epigastric pain, stridor, hoarseness of voice, coughing, respiratory distress points toward severe injury:
- Stridor, hoarseness of voice, coughing, respiratory distress: Laryngeal/tracheal involvement.
- Odynophagia, drooling of saliva: Moderate/severe involvement of oral cavity.
- Dysphagia is due to esophageal injury and edema
- History of sudden chest pain after consumption points toward thoracic esophageal perforation
- History of severe epigastric pain points toward gastric perforation
- Hematemesis points toward ulcers/full thickness perforation or rarely to aorto-enteric fistula in which case it is fatal

3. *Treatment received for the immediate insult*:
   - History of intubation and/or tracheostomy: Points toward severe injury and/or respiratory involvement.
   - History of treatment on OPD basis suggests mild disease whereas admission in ward suggests significant injury, while admission to ICU suggests even more severe injury leading to perforation, bleeding.
   - Details regarding endoscopic evaluation: It is usually done within first 2-3 days of consumption and is prohibited between days 5-15 (due to increased risk of perforation). Performed to grade the severity of the injury as per Zargar classification and to manage accordingly **(Table 1)**
   - Alkali consumption—3 phases of liquefactive necrosis:
     - Acute (up to 3 days)
     - Ulceration and granulation (3 days to 3 weeks: weakest phase)
     - Cicatrization and stricture formation (3 weeks to 3 months)
     - Stricture stabilization takes up to 6-12 months, so surgery is best done after 12 months, especially in pharyngeal strictures

     Nasogastric or nasojejunal tube placement is not recommended as it may by itself lead to long stricture formation.

     However, if nasogastric or nasojejunal tube has already been inserted somewhere else, then it may be used for enteral nutrition (immediate) and dilatation over it (later).

     A feeding jejunostomy is the recommended method to facilitate enteral nutrition. Note, when was it performed and how many calories the patient has been receiving per day.

     (Feeding gastrostomy must be avoided as stomach then cannot be used as conduit if required)

TABLE 1: Zargar classification		
Grade	**Description**	**Management**
Grade 1	Only erythema and edema	(Heals without stricture)
Grade 2a	Superficial erosions	
Grade 2b	Deep and/or circumferential ulcers	(Heals with stricture)
Grade 3a	Scattered areas of necrosis	
Grade 3b	Extensive necrosis	(Needs surgery: Esophagectomy needed as primary repair is not possible as the tissue is unhealthy)
Grade 4	Perforation	

4. *Course of the injury over the months*:
   - History of postprandial heaviness, nausea, vomiting: Suggests gastric outlet obstruction due to corrosive gastric stricture (*PARTIAL GASTRIC involvement*)
   - History of early satiety: Suggests extensive gastric cicatrization (*COMPLETE GASTRIC involvement*)
   - History of colicky abdominal pain, abdominal distention, ball rolling sensation, nausea, vomiting, borborygmi (*DUODENUM and SMALL BOWEL involvement*)
     - Treatment history for dysphagia: History of contrast studies/cross-sectional imaging/endoscopy
     - History of dilatation therapy: Note when it was started, the number of sessions and total duration of therapy
5. *Past history—History of psychiatric illness/previous suicidal tendencies*:
   - To know compliance to treatment
6. *History of pulmonary diseases* like bronchial asthma and chronic obstructive pulmonary disease to plan for respiratory optimization before surgery
7. *Personal history—Smoking history*: To anticipate delayed weaning off ventilator/delayed wound healing
8. *Performance status*: For treatment planning/prehabilitation

EXAMINATION PROFORMA

On a preliminary survey, Look out for:
- Patients carrying a spittoon with them, into which they spit even their saliva every few minutes as they are suffering from complete dysphagia
- Nasogastric/nasojejunal or feeding jejunostomy tube in situ
- Surgical scars in neck, chest or abdomen

General Examination: Part A

- *Visual appearance*:
  - Young/middle aged/elderly
- *Gender*:
  - Male/female
- *Built*: Poor/average/good
- *Nourishment*: Poor/average/good
- *Poor nourishment features*:
  - Temporal wasting
  - Sunken eyes
  - Flattened cheeks, Buccal hollow
  - Supraclavicular hollow
  - Squaring of shoulders
  - Prominent scapula
  - Prominent intercostal spaces
  - Scaphoid abdomen
  - Prominent hip bones

- Prominent knees and elbows
- Pedal edema
- Decreased mid-arm circumference
- Decreased skinfold thickness
- Measure height, weight, BMI
- Mention regarding feeding access—enteral/parenteral or both

Clinical evaluation:
- Conscious/stuporous
- Cooperative/uncooperative
- Orientation to time, place and person: Present/absent
- Hydration status: Hydrated/dehydrated
- Lying comfortably in bed/in discomfort/in pain
- Whether patient prefers sitting or lying down position
- Febrile/Afebrile

Vitals: Pulse, BP, respiratory rate, mention performance status here as well

General Examination: Part B

- *Look for PICCLE, skin (previous suicidal cuts), oral cavity, neck, chest, abdomen (scars/peristalsis)*: Pallor, icterus, cyanosis, clubbing, generalized or localized lymphadenopathy, palpable cervical and left supraclavicular lymph node, pedal or dependent edema
- *Examination of oral cavity*:
    - Restricted mouth opening/tongue movement due to scarring
    - Look for erythema, edema, discoloration of mucosa, ulcer, slough, eschar
- *Examination of the neck*: For scar of previous cervical exploration (for management of complex pharyngeal strictures—to allow retrograde dilatation of the stricture over guidewire: Professor Anantakrishnan's technique) or of diversion cervical esophagostomy, for esophageal perforation.

Abdominal Examination

Look for the presence of any feeding jejunostomy (FJ) which may be done for feeding access in cases of complete dysphagia.

On inspection, see if:
- Abdominal contour: Flat/distended/scaphoid
- Umbilicus: Central/displaced. Inverted/everted/flat
- All quadrants are moving equally with respiration or not
- Look for surgical scars of previous surgery done for luminal perforation secondary to corrosive injury.
- Look for visible gastric peristalsis (from left to right) which will be seen in gastric corrosive injury leading to gastric outlet obstruction.
- Look for visible lump, sinus, engorged veins, pulsations or cough impulse.
- Inspect the groin hernial sites and genitalia.
- Inspection of renal angles to look for fullness

On palpation, see if:
- Abdomen is soft and nontender
- Liver is palpable or not
- Spleen is enlarged or not
- Any other palpable lump
- Palpate groin hernia sites and examine genitals
- Look for tenderness in renal angles
- Examine back and spine

On percussion:
- Look for upper border of liver dullness (generally in the 5th intercostal space) in midclavicular line.
- Note the liver span (normal being 12–14 cm)
- Percussion note in the rest of the abdomen (generally tympanic)
- Tests for free fluid

On auscultation:
- Auscultate for bowel sounds
- Bruit, hum and rub
- Per-rectal examination

Respiratory Examination

Inspection:
- Tracheal position: Midline/deviated
- Bilateral chest movement—equal or not

Palpation:
- Trachea central or deviated
- Bilateral chest movement—equal or not
- Chest, look for warmth and tenderness
- Tactile vocal fremitus—it is increased in case of pleural effusion and consolidation.

Percussion:
- Normal percussion note is resonant.
- Dull note suggests consolidation or pleural effusion.

Auscultation:
Breath sounds
- Bilaterally—equal or not
- Reduced breath sounds would suggest either pleural effusion or consolidation

Adventitious sounds
- Crepts—coarse crepts would suggest aspiration pneumonitis, whereas fine crepts would suggest pulmonary edema.
- Rhonchi/wheeze

    So just remember that increased TVF, Dull note and reduced breath sounds = Effusion/Consolidation

Rest systemic examination

MANAGEMENT

Emergency Management of Corrosive Consumption Injury

Examine oral cavity, vocal cords, airways—if any need for intubation or do emergency tracheostomy, if there is severe laryngeal injury. Simultaneously assess circulation, vitals, resuscitate with IV fluids, start inotropes if needed, send baseline investigations (BLI) as follows: Hemogram, electrolytes, renal and liver function tests. Start broad spectrum antibiotics.

Examine chest and abdomen to rule out subcutaneous emphysema, abdominal tenderness signifying perforation, and after patient stable, get chest X-ray (CXR), abdominal X-ray (AXR) done to rule out hydropneumothorax and gas under diaphragm. If positive, get a CECT done, if patient stable and shift to OT, do esophagectomy/gastrectomy with proximal esophagostomy, FJ and come out. Do reconstruction at a later date.

If no perforation on clinical evaluation, then after corrosive consumption, upper GI endoscopy (UGIE) best done between 48-72 hours to grade the injury as per Zargars classification and to see if stomach/duodenum is affected. Avoid UGIE between 5-15 days as high risk of perforation.

Zargars Grades of Injury along with their Management

Grade 1: Erythema, edema
Grade 2a: Focal ulcers
Grade 2b: Circumferential ulcers
Grade 3a: Focal necrosis
Grade 3b: Extensive necrosis
Grade 4: Perforation

Grade 1, 2a: Conservative management, start orals, discharge—healing without strictures
Grade 2b, 3a: Nil per oral (NPO), IV fluids, antibiotics, monitor, will heal with strictures and hence, need FJ for feeding access in the same admission, followed by endoscopic dilatation starting after 3 weeks.
Grade 3b, 4: Emergency surgery (Esophagectomy only. No primary repair as tissue is unhealthy)

Three Phases of Injury after Alkali Consumption

1. *Acute phase*: Within 3 days
2. *Phase of ulceration and granulation*: 3 days to 3 weeks (Weakest phase)
3. *Phase of cicatrization and stricture formation*: 3 weeks to 3 months.

Stricture starts forming after 3 weeks and progresses rapidly. Gastric, esophageal and pharyngoesophageal strictures stabilize at 3, 6 and 12 months respectively. Hence, endoscopic dilatation must be started immediately after 3 weeks otherwise there will be complete obliteration of lumen. Whereas for surgery, it is best to wait up to 12 months for the stricture to completely stabilize.

After corrosive injury, Ryles tube/nasojejunal tube (NJ) should not be placed because if placed blindly, can convert partial injury to full perforation, can itself lead to a long stricture formation due to persistent reflux across gastroesophageal junction (GEJ).

However, if it has been placed somewhere else, it can be used for feeding and then dilatation over it can be done, but it should be removed early, while dilatation should be continued till patient is ready for surgery (ideally after 12 months).

So if patient presents on day 5 after ingestion, UGIE is contraindicated. Do not do barium as well (risk of mediastinitis), Just do FJ.

Then after 3 weeks, do barium and UGIE and manage with dilatation up to 6-12 months till stricture stabilizes.

FJ is the procedure of choice for feeding access in these patients who develop dysphagia and strictures.

Principles of Endoscopic Dilatation

1. Started after 3 weeks (as before that, chance of perforation is high) and not to wait beyond that, as strictures progress fast.
2. Savary-Gilliard is preferred over balloon, as longer strictures can be longitudinally as well as radially dilated. Balloon has only radial force and so has more chance of perforation.
3. At each dilatation, not more than 3 consecutive dilators should be used, for a max dilatation of 3F (1F = 0.33 mm). Sessions done every 2 weeks, till ≥14 mm lumen is reached.
4. Fully-covered self-expandable metal stent (FC-SEMS)/Biodegradable stents can be used for long-term dilatation (for nutrition and can avoid need for surgery as well)

Indications of Surgery

- Stricture >10 cm
- >3 strictures
- Stricture associated with proximal diverticulum (high risk of perforation)
- Past history of perforation after dilatation
- *Refractory stricture*: >5 sessions done at 2 week intervals, but not able to dilate to 14 mm
- *Recurrent stricture*: Not able to maintain lumen of 14 mm, 4 weeks after successful dilatation.

Stricture takes 6-12 months to mature, so surgery for stricture is best done after 12 months.

Risk of Malignancy in Esophageal Stricture

Very less, max up to 2% (mostly seen with alkaline consumption after 30-40 years latency, whereas in India we see more of acid consumption), hence bypass preferred to resection, as if risk of cancer was more, then endoscopic dilatation would not have been the initial accepted treatment and sometimes even the definitive treatment.

Repeated trauma caused by dilatation itself can actually increase the risk of *MALIGNANCY*.

Advantages of Resection (Though not Advisable)
- Eliminates malignancy
- Posterior mediastinal route can be used for conduit, which is shortest (30 cm) and more physiological
- Native esophageal dilatation and esophagocele is prevented

So Evaluation of Patient of Corrosive Stricture Referred to You
1. Review old records along with treatment done, route of nutrition
2. Do CXR first to see lung changes (patchy infiltrates due to aspiration/consolidation/effusion), followed by indirect laryngoscopy and hypopharyngoscopy to assess posterior pharyngeal wall, pyriform sinus, epiglottis, vocal cords and to break any synechiae if present
3. Then do barium esophagogram to see location—how far from upper esophageal sphincter (UES)/length/number of strictures/their morphology, any diverticulum proximal to the stricture, if stomach/duodenum involved (any stricture/growth seen)
4. Then do UGIE to assess same things + see for any other lesions/stasis esophagitis/ulcers and biopsy if any suspicious lesion/irregular looking stricture
5. Then CECT oral and IV contrast to assess pulmonary complications, then to have a roadmap, to assess stricture morphology (whether uniform and smooth OR irregular with shouldering), to assess stomach (whether any stricture/growth) and to assess colonic vascular anatomy/arterial stenosis (in old patients, or previously operated patients) (in preparation for conduit use)
6. *Grade pharyngoesophageal strictures*: 6 types **(Table 2)**
7. *Grade gastric strictures*: 7 types **(Table 3)**
8. Do full length colonoscopy (for colon conduit evaluation)

TABLE 2: Pharyngoesophageal corrosive strictures classification[1]	
PES: Severity classification	
Group	**Findings**
Group I	Residual lumen capable of admitting a guidewire
Group II	No demonstrable lumen obviating passage of a guidewire: Extreme proximity of the stricture to the laryngeal inlet leading to respiratory embarrassment
Group III	Short segment PES due to granulation tissue or synechiae
Group IV	Dense nondilatable stricture of the pharyngoesophageal (PE) junction with a normal distal esophagus at least 5 cm length distal to pharyngoesophageal stricture (PES)
Group V	Total destruction of the larynx
Group VI	No lumen was detected in the cervical esophageal segment beyond the PES by contrast study or CT scan

TABLE 3: Isolated corrosive gastric strictures classification[2]	
Type	Location of Stricture in Stomach
Type I	Stricture <5 cm from pyloroduodenal ring
Type II	Stricture >5 cm from pyloroduodenal ring
Type IIA	Stricture <1 cm
Type III	Stricture >1 cm
Type IV	Mid body stricture
Type V	Diffuse gastric stricture
Type V	Proximal or gastroesophageal junction stricture
Type VI	Digital gastric stricture involving duodenum
Type VII	Double stricture (gastroesophageal junction and antrum)

Note: Isolated corrosive gastric strictures:
- New Working Classification and Management Strategies
- SSAT Annual Meeting 2015

9. See all blood reports, especially albumin. Optimization of nutrition (end points: Weight gain, BMI and albumin) with FJ if needed (at least for 6 weeks before definitive surgery), with psychiatric consultation
10. Plan management accordingly.

Before Surgery

Give full bowel preparation.

Remember, for a high (pharyngeal) anastomosis, neck should be explored first, bimanual palpation of pharynx should be done with one finger inside mouth and another through the incision, to check if it is healthy and not fibrosed. Only then proceed to abdomen for mobilizing conduit.

As a rule, anastomosis is best done below the UES, to the cervical esophagus, because if done above UES, it leads to severe aspiration and pulmonary morbidity as it is very difficult to learn swallowing with a pharyngeal anastomosis.

Now if Cervical Esophagus is not Available for Anastomosis, then Three Options

1. Try to create a neoesophagus (just below the UES) with myocutaneous flaps (sternomastoid/pectoralis/intercostal) and then coloplasty can be done to the neoesophagus; OR
2. Pharyngocoloplasty with a permanent tracheostomy (because there's profound reflux and aspiration, as it is very difficult to learn to swallow without aspirating, with a pharyngeal anastomosis, as it is above the UES); OR
3. Make a permanent FJ (if patient not willing for permanent tracheostomy as quality of life (QOL) with FJ is better than a pharyngeal anastomosis without a tracheostomy).

Hence, all attempts must be made preoperatively to dilate the stricture to be able to anastomose below the UES.

Also, *for esophageal corrosive strictures, always a bypass is done* (with colon/jejunum/stomach) as resection is risky due to dense periesophageal adhesions and minimal cancer risk, and all proximal anastomoses are done in the neck.

Few Exceptions in which Resection is Done

1. For a short segment distal esophageal corrosive/peptic stricture, for which short segment resection and replacement with a jejunal interposition conduit can be done.
2. If there is a segment of esophagus cut-off proximally and distally due to strictures at both ends, then esophagectomy can be done to prevent esophagocele (mucus collection).
3. In pediatric patients, esophagectomy should be attempted as longer duration may predispose to cancer.

Also, before planning for esophageal bypass, stomach should be evaluated and accordingly, it must be decided where to anastomose the lower end of conduit (to stomach OR to Roux-en-Y loop of jejunum).

If Along with Esophagus

1. Only pylorus and prepyloric region is strictured, then do segmental resection of that part with a Billroth-1 reconstruction, and then do esophagocoloplasty, and distal end of colon anastomose to upper part of remnant stomach.
2. Distal stomach is involved, but with healthy D1 then do distal gastrectomy followed by reconstruction with GJ (Loop/Roux-en-Y) and then do esophagocoloplasty, and distal end of colon anastomosis to upper remnant stomach.
3. *Distal stomach and D1 both involved, then only do* GJ (Loop/Roux-en-Y), as an affected D1 will be a difficult duodenum to close after gastrectomy, and will lead to stump blowout. And then do esophagocoloplasty, and distal end of colon anastomose to stomach.
4. Full stomach is involved but with healthy D1, then do total gastrectomy, and then do esophagocoloplasty and distal end of colon anastomose to Roux-en-Y loop of jejunum (Roux-en-Y is preferred to loop, as bile reflux into colon can cause colonic CA).
5. *Entire stomach and D1 both involved*, then do esophagocoloplasty and distal end of colon anastomose to Roux loop of jejunum.

If esophagus is normal and only stomach is affected then do segmental/distal/total gastrectomy.

But if distal stomach and D1 both involved, then just do a GJ (for above mentioned reasons).

And if entire stomach and D1 both involved, then just bypass stomach and D1 with Roux-en-Y EJ.

So COLON is the Best Conduit for Corrosive Strictures for the Following Reasons

1. Better than jejunum as it allows more length.
2. Better than stomach, because no acid reflux, no secondary peptic stricture, and will always be unaffected by corrosives. However, more complex procedure, requires complete colonoscopy and colon vascular evaluation by CT angio before surgery. Colonic diverticulosis/polyposis/lesions or colonic vessel atheromas contraindicate it's use as conduit.

Situations for Jejunum as a Conduit

1. Just remember that for a *short segment distal* esophageal corrosive/peptic stricture, resection and replacement with a jejunal interposition conduit (based on native supply) can be done. So in that, End-to-side (ES) esophagojejunostomy (EJ) is done proximally and ES jejunogastrostomy (JG) is done distally with anterior stomach.
2. Also, if colon and stomach, both are not available for various issues, then even for a complete esophageal bypass requiring a neck anastomosis, a jejunal free graft (not based on native supply, but supercharged with internal thyroid artery or internal mammary artery) may be used.

Types of Colon Conduit

Right colon [based on middle colic artery (MCA)], left colon [based on ascending branch of left colic artery (LCA)] and middle colon/modified left colon (again based on ascending branch of LCA)—Professor Ananthkrishnan and Professor Kate group.

Advantages of right colon—better lumen match of ileum with esophagus, and less reflux due to IC valve, but variable vascular anatomy (RCA present in only 30%), so higher chance of conduit ischemia, necrosis, leak, fistula and later on stricture.

Advantages of left colon—less bulky, wall thickness comparable with esophagus, and has dependable vascular anatomy.

However, right and left coloplasties—fixed length, causing more tension on anastomosis and more chance of ischemia, necrosis, leak. Can measure length of conduit from IMA root to angle of mandible to see if it's adequate.

Hence, *the idea of modified left colon conduit* (by Professor Ananthkrishnan and Professor Kate group), so ileum transected 2 cm proximal to IC, up to mid descending colon, pulled up to neck by ileum, so no traction on colonic vascular arcade, and after getting it in neck, redundant ileum and ascending colon are shaved off. So it always has a comfortable length, no tension, and dependable blood supply and is to be preferred.

Before anastomosis, the xiphoid can be resected so that pressure on conduit is reduced. If venous congestion is still seen, then thoracic inlet has to be widened by resecting left clavicular head/medial half of 1st two ribs/left half of manubrium sterni: Be careful of brachiocephalic trunk. If arterial supply looks compromised, then arcade can be supercharged with inferior thyroid artery or internal mammary artery OR conduit may have to be changed (So if it is right colon, then instead use left colon/modified left colon).

Side-to-side (SS) esophagocolonic anastomosis (hand sewn single layered, interrupted, with absorbable sutures OR linear stapler for SS, done in the neck) is best as generally the tip of the conduit has less blood supply/is ischemic, so doing a SS helps to avoid the ischemic tip while getting a well vascularized segment, and also a wide 5 cm anastomosis can be made, decreasing chance of stricture, and even if that happens, it can be easily dilated. Also SS helps prevent mucocele of remnant esophagus as doing an ES anastomosis will create a closed compartment of esophageal segment between the upper cut and sealed end, and the stricture lower down, leading to esophagocele.

Always add FJ after esophageal bypass, and if any FG was made previously, close it.

If in immediate postoperative period there is fever, tachycardia, lactic acidosis, suspect conduit ischemia/necrosis. Immediately open neck wound to assess esophagocolic/esophagogastric/esophagojejunal anastomosis and visually inspect for ischemia/necrosis. Resuscitate, shift for emergency UGIE by an expert with minimal air insufflation and get CECT done to see if it's partial/full thickness ischemia.

If partial ischemia, then debride that part of conduit and reanastomose, buttress with sternocleidomastoid flap. But if the entire conduit is gangrenous, then resect conduit, do proximal esophagostomy, give wide drainage and come out and do bypass later (opposite colon or jejunum can be used as conduit).

In the meantime continue FJ feeds.

■ REFERENCES

1. Ananthakrishnan N, Kate V, Parthasarathy G. Therapeutic options for management of pharyngoesophageal corrosive strictures. J Gastrointest Surg. 2011;15:566-75.
2. Manickavasagam K, Chandramohan A, Devigounder K, Murugesan CS. Mo1677 Isolated Corrosive Gastric Strictures-New Working Classification and Management Strategies. Gastroenterology. 2015;148(4):S-1170.

2.3 CHAPTER

Upper Gastrointestinal—Ward

Few clinical tips and management of a few commonly encountered complications which will help you in ward rounds.

■ MEDICAL MANAGEMENT OF VARICEAL BLEED

- *Terlipressin*: 0.2–2 mg IV QID for 5 days
- *Octreotide*: 100 mics bolus followed by 50 mics/hour infusion
- With antibiotics, and albumin infusion

■ CASE OF BILIOUS VOMITING

So if vomiting is multiple times without abdominal distention, then it is likely to be proximal complete small bowel obstruction (SBO) due to extramural pathology, like adhesive band obstruction. But if frequency is less, then it is likely due to partial SBO due to partial lumen occlusion due to intramural growth. Remember any lesion can present both ways. And in cases of bilious vomiting without any other positive features, always consider Wilkies syndrome. And if there is pain in abdomen, with distention, visible peristalsis, then most likely it is distal SBO.

Any postoperative complication, first assess the complete picture, what it is most likely to be, then go step-by-step from basic tests to advanced.

■ MANAGEMENT OF ESOPHAGEAL PERFORATION AND POST-ESOPHAGECTOMY RELATED COMPLICATIONS

Management of Esophageal Perforation

Do contrast-enhanced computed tomography (CECT) with intravenous (IV) and oral water soluble contrast or esophagogram (water soluble): If contained perforation (caused by instrument) with contrast draining back into lumen and minimal sepsis, and non-diseased esophagus, manage conservatively with nil per oral (NPO), IV fluids, antibiotics, total parenteral nutrition (TPN).

If free perforation:
- *Good performance status*: Surgery
  - Healthy tissue in non diseased esophagus (generally <24 hours):
    - Primary closure
  - Same in diseased esophagus (end-stage achalasia, stricture, cancer):
    - Esophagectomy
  - Unhealthy tissue (generally >24 hours):
    - Exclusion of perforation (proximal diversion by esophagostomy and distally stapled), pleural space drainage, venting gastrostomy and feeding jejunostomy (FJ).
- *Poor performance status*:
  - Endoscopic treatment: OTSC (over the scope clips), endosuture, fully covered self-expandable metal stents (FC-SEMS), with pleural drainage.
  - If success—remove stent after 6 weeks.
  - If ongoing sepsis—surgery

Just an interesting point to note: Remember that by postoperative day 5 (POD5), in 97% there is no postoperative gas under diaphragm. So any significant gas under diaphragm after POD5, is perforation.

MANAGEMENT OF TRACHEOBRONCHIAL TEAR DURING TRANSHIATAL ESOPHAGECTOMY (THE)

- If patient stable—complete the THE, and pull up gastric tube as a very small leak will seal off.
- If unstable (large air leak), tell anesthetist to deflate cuff, advance it beyond tear, reinflate and do single lung ventilation.
- Then do right posterolateral thoracotomy
  - <1 cm: Simple closure with polydioxanone suture (PDS), buttress with conduit
  - >1 cm: Closure and then buttress with vascularized pedicle (intercostal flap)

THE FOLLOWING SECTION IS ABOUT POSTOPERATIVE ESOPHAGEAL ANASTOMOSES ISSUES AND THEIR MANAGEMENT

Use these same principles for issues after esophageal anastomoses done for any indication, whether after resection of esophagus (as for perforation/cancer) or bypass (as for corrosive stricture).

So post-anastomoses, collections can be due to:
- Anastomotic leak (bile and enteric contents)
- Lymphorrhea [after extensive lymph node (LN) dissection]
- Chyle leak (seen after thoracic duct injury)
- If dissection very close to pancreas, then pancreatic leak from small ducts/main pancreatic duct (MPD) leading to pure pancreatic leak

- Inflammatory collection
- Postoperative surgical site fluid (seen after most cases)

Esophageal anastomosis leak types by Lerut:
- *Radiological*: No symptoms/signs, purely radiological diagnosis
- *Clinical minor*: Fever/Leukocytosis, cervical wound inflammation/drainage (without ischemia/necrosis of conduit and without systemic sepsis) or a contained thoracic leak
- *Clinical major*: Minor disruption, but leading to systemic sepsis or major disruption needing surgical revision
- *Conduit necrosis*: Needing esophageal resection/diversion

Endoscopic interventions:
- OTSC
- Overstitch
- Endoscopic vacuum therapy [polyurethane sponge within cavity or lumen. Nasogastric tube (NGT) connects this to low pressure vacuum −100 to −125 mm Hg. Sponge changed every 3 days for cavitary and weekly for luminal]
- FC-SEMS

Surgical indications:
- Early leak <72 hours
- Failed conservative/endoscopic management
- Severe sepsis

So management of cervical anastomosis leak as per various situations:
- *Asymptomatic/Minimally symptomatic:*
  - Open cervical wound and clean with isotonic fluid
  - NPO
  - Feed via FJ
  - +− Antibiotics
  - +− NGT
  - +− Intercostal drainage tube (ICD) for pleura/mediastinum
- *Symptomatic with local (neck) inflammation:*
  - All of the above, + antibiotics, NGT, ICD
- *Early leak without ischemia:*
  - Preserve conduit
  - Suture the defects, buttress with sternocleidomastoid flap
- *Early leak with local ischemia:*
  - Resection of ischemic area with re-anastomosis, buttress with muscle flap.
- *Severe sepsis/necrosis:*
  - Conduit resection with cervical esophagostomy

So management of thoracic anastomosis leak as per various situations:
- *Asymptomatic/Minimally symptomatic:*
  - NPO
  - NGT
  - Feed via FJ

- Antibiotics
- +– ICD for pleura/mediastinum
- *Symptomatic with controlled sepsis*:
  - ICD + endoscopic interventions
- *Early leak without/with local ischemia*:
  - Thoracotomy, washing, drainage
  - Resection of ischemic area with re-anastomosis, buttress with muscle flap.
- *Severe sepsis/necrosis*:
  - Conduit resection with cervical esophagostomy

Chyle Leak

Bed side test:
- Dissolves in ether
- Give oral fat with methylene blue, and see chest drain

Biochemical tests:
- Triglycerides >110 mg/dL
- Cholesterol <200 mg/dL
- High number of lymphocytes

Microscopy: Chylomicrons are seen.

Chyle composition: Proteins, fats, sugars, electrolytes, albumin, globulin, fibrinogen, prothrombin, antithrombin, lymphocytes and RBCs.

Complications of routine thoracic duct ligation: Retroperitoneal and pedal edema, nutritional and immunological adverse effects. And leak can still happen because of variant anatomy.

Management of Chyle Leak

Conservative first, fat free diet/start medium chain triglycerides (MCTs), drain pleural space if required. If no response, keep NPO, start IV fluids, TPN. If no response, start octreotide/etilefrine (smooth muscle agonist), try pleurodesis.

If after this output is on falling trend, and goes below 250 mL/day, then restart diet with MCT (coconut oil), low fats and high protein. If drainage stops, remove drain. But if trend again goes up after starting diet, plan intervention.

Other Indications for Intervention

If after maximal conservative, medical therapy and pleurodesis:
- >1.5 L in 48 hours, or
- >500 mL after >5 days, or
- <500 after 14 days (same trend)

Then two options: Interventional radiology (IR) or surgery.
1. *Interventional radiology*:
   - Lymphangioscintigraphy can be done (web spaces of foot/inguinal nodes-lipiodol) to localize. Then CT guided embolization done, via cisterna chyli, using super selective catheters.

2. *Surgery*:
   - Indocyanine green (ICG) can be used, 0.5 mg/kg in bilateral inguinal nodes—1 hour before surgery or fat/methylene blue given via Ryles tube on table.
   - Then find leak point and ligate or do supradiaphragmatic mass ligation between azygos and aorta.

■ POST-GASTROJEJUNOSTOMY CLINICAL ISSUES

- *Persistent high output Ryles tube (gastric contents)*:
  ○ Can be due to Stomal edema, Stomal narrowing
- *Persistent high output Ryles tube (bilious)*:
  ○ Can be delayed gastric emptying (DGE) due to gastroparesis or atony or ileus or due to efferent loop block

Treatment: First rule out obstruction with CECT with oral contrast and upper gastrointestinal endoscopy (UGIE). If efferent loop block, go for surgery to correct kink, hernia.

If no block, then correct electrolytes, sugars, start feeding jejunostomy (FJ)/nasojejunal (NJ) feeds, prokinetics, or gastric pacemaker.

If persistent high output even after 4–6 weeks then last resort is gastrectomy (distal/near total) with revision anastomosis. Counsel that roux loop stasis may again lead to similar problems but will settle.

■ POST-GASTRECTOMY ISSUES AND RELATED CLINICAL COMPLICATIONS

If proximal margin comes positive for malignancy, then two options:
1. If patient fit, biopsy is well-moderately differentiated, and very few LN are + even after adequate LN dissection, then go in for re-resection.
2. However, if patient unfit or biopsy is poorly differentiated or multiple dissected nodes +, then go for adjuvant chemoradiotherapy (CRT).

Also, do immunohistochemistry (IHC) for HER2/neu, microsatellite instability (MSI), PD-L1. So if +, add trastuzumab based on TOGA trial, and if MSI-H or deficient, then add PD-L1 inhibitor like pembrolizumab (keynote trial) or nivolumab (checkmate trial).

Also if MSI high in preoperative biopsy, then it would not be respond to 5-FU chemo and add oxaliplatin in adjuvant.

After total gastrectomy and Roux-en-Y esophagojejunostomy (EJ) with jejunojejunostomy (JJ), orals can be started once ileus resolves after day 3, for which RT output is documented. If high even after day 3 (>500), see vitals, see drains, send all baseline investigations (BLI). Causes for it are:
- Persistent ileus, or
- Obstruction distal to EJ, or at JJ site, or beyond JJ at FJ site, or beyond FJ.

Now if vitally unstable and drains show bile, first suspect duodenal blowout or leak at EJ or JJ or FJ site.

For blowout: Resuscitate, send BLI, do USG and drain collections, CECT with oral contrast to know site, if leak seen, go in early, lavage, if kink at FJ, repair it, also try to repair JJ or EJ if tissue healthy, otherwise just put drains and give FJ feeds in postoperative period.

■ DUODENAL INJURY REPAIR (OUR TECHNIQUE WHICH HAS HELPED SALVAGE PATIENTS OF DUODENAL INJURY REFERRED TO US)

Ensure ryles tube is in place, in the stomach. Then ask for a Frekas (Nasojejunal tube) and push it beyond the injury.

Debride the edges of the injury if unhealthy. Plan to close it perpendicular to the long axis of duodenum. Take and tie corner Connell sutures at both corners. Then start from the farthest end. Use interrupted Connell sutures for closure. (After taking one Connell throw on both sides, thread is pulled up and suture is tied. This is continued till the other corner is reached). If possible, take a second layer of lembert. If NJ tube could not be manipulated distal to injury, add a duodenostomy distal to the closure, from the duodenal segment closest to the abdominal wall. Take prolene purse string to fix the duodenostomy tube on the duodenal side. Then fix it like how a drain is fixed on the abdominal skin side. Then add an FJ. Then place a Morrison drain, pelvic drain from opposite side and a subcutaneous drain. Subcutaneous drain helps to drain any intra-abdominal collection which may collect in the subcutaneous space in case of a small dehiscence.

3.1 CHAPTER

Hepatopancreatobiliary: Malignant Surgical Obstructive Jaundice— History/Examination Discussion

■ HISTORY

- *Onset of jaundice*: Insidious onset is seen due to malignant pathology whereas relatively sudden onset jaundice is seen in benign causes of obstructive jaundice (OJ) like biliary stone disease and rare causes like hemobilia after blunt trauma abdomen or after any biliary tree intervention (endoscopic/surgical)
- *Duration of jaundice*: Short in malignant causes (few weeks). Long duration is seen in benign causes (biliary stone disease or choledochal cyst).
- *Nature of jaundice*:
  - *Progressive*: Gradually deepening. Hallmark of malignant etiology—carcinoma HOP, carcinoma gallbladder or perihilar cholangiocarcinoma. Exception being benign biliary stricture (BBS) which is likely the only benign entity cause causing progressive obstructive jaundice.
  - *Fluctuating*: Bilirubin levels do not normalize but keep waxing and waning. Hallmark of periampullary cancers—initially tumor completely obstructs the biliary outflow leading to rapid rise in bilirubin levels, however when the tumor sloughs off, the obstruction becomes partial and the bilirubin levels drop, but not completely. Tumor sloughing off can lead to bleeding presenting as melena.
  - *Intermittent*: Bilirubin levels normalize between two episodes of hyperbilirubinemia. Seen in benign pathology like biliary stone disease and hemobilia (bilirubin normalizes after the stone or clot has been passed).
  - Presence of prodromal symptoms (nausea, vomiting, myalgia, malaise) is seen in medical causes of jaundice like viral hepatitis.
- *History of pain*:
  - Benign causes: Biliary stone disease, cholangitis
  - Malignant causes: Head of pancreas (HOP) cancer, gallbladder cancer (GBC)
  - Site: Right hypochondrium and epigastrium +/− radiation to mid back or right infrascapular region

- Onset: Pain in biliary stone disease is usually sudden in onset, whereas pain in malignancy is insidious in onset.
- Duration: Short in malignant causes (few weeks). Long duration is seen in benign causes (biliary stone disease or choledochal cyst).
- Nature: Intermittent (biliary stone disease or choledochal cyst)/continuous (malignant diseases)/progressive (benign-chronic pancreatitis; malignant-pancreatic and GBC)
- Character: Dull aching in malignant causes whereas colicky in biliary stone disease or choledochal cyst
- Intensity: Mild/moderate/severe—to know whether quality of life (QOL) impaired.
- Postprandial association: Seen in pancreatobiliary pathology.
- Postural association: Reduction in pain on bending forwards suggests pancreatic pathology.
- Recent change in nature of pain in chronic pancreatitis—from intermittent to continuous/progressive is a harbinger of malignancy in background of long-standing chronic pancreatitis.
- *History of pruritus*: Pruritus in a jaundiced patient suggests obstructive pathology. Etiology being endogenous opioids, serotonin. Severe pruritus affecting QOL, itself is an indication for biliary drainage. (Patients may become suicidal due to unrelenting pruritus and needs to be addressed in an expedited fashion in such a case.)
- *Color of stools (cholic or acholic) and urine (high colored)*:
  - Passage of clay colored stools and high colored urine in a jaundiced patient suggests complete obstruction to flow of bile from bile duct into the intestinal lumen, whereas passage of cholic stools (usual brown colored) suggests partial/no obstruction to flow of bile.
  - Passage of clay colored stools in a jaundiced patient suggests complete biliary obstruction, while pruritus may be present even with partial obstruction.
  - Also remember that intrahepatic cholestatic phase of medical jaundice can also present similarly (transient presentation)
- *History suggestive of fat-soluble vitamin deficiency*: Due to long-term fat malabsorption. Night blindness (vitamin A), osteomalacia leading to fractures (vitamin D), male infertility (vitamin E) and hemorrhage (vitamin K). Generally seen in benign causes due to longer duration
- *History to rule out chronic liver disease*:
  - Abdominal distension due to ascites
  - GI bleed due to variceal bleed
  - Altered sensorium due to hepatic encephalopathy
  - Infections, bleeding tendencies due to symptomatic hypersplenism
- *History of fever*: Points towards cholangitis. Generally seen in benign causes. However, periampullary cancer violates the sphincter and may present with cholangitis without any biliary interventions. Biliary interventions like stent placement [plastic more often than self-expandable metal stent (SEMS)] predisposes the patient to cholangitis

- *History of postprandial upper abdominal heaviness, nausea, voluminous nonbilious vomiting containing partially digested food* suggests gastric outlet obstruction (GOO). Generally seen in patients with carcinoma HOP, locally advanced GBC and chronic pancreatitis associated with head mass (inflammatory or malignant)
- *History of hematemesis or melena*: May be seen in periampullary cancer due to tumor sloughing off periodically due to necrosis and even in head of pancreas cancer (HOP CA) and GBC infiltrating duodenum.
- *History of postural dizziness, syncope, fatigue, shortness of breath, need for blood transfusion*: To know the severity of blood loss and to plan for management—whether only blood transfusions or angioembolization or hemostatic radiotherapy (RT) or expedited surgery.
- *History of recent onset diabetes above 50 years of age flags the onset of pancreatic cancer*. Worsening of glycemic control in previously well controlled type 2 diabetes or in type 3C chronic pancreatitis also flags the onset of pancreatic cancer.
- *History of loss of weight (LOW), loss of appetite (LOA)*:
  - Beware: LOW happens in benign (chronic pancreatitis) as well as malignant causes, however LOA happens with malignancy only
- *History of metastatic disease*:
  - Abdominal distension: Due to malignant ascites
  - Dry cough, hemoptysis: Due to pleural effusion and lung metastasis
  - Bony pain, nontraumatic fractures: Due to bony metastasis
  - Unexplained sudden new onset headaches, blackouts, seizures: Due to brain metastasis
- *Treatment history*: History of ERC and endoscopic biliary stenting, or endoscopically placed nasal tube (ENBD) or percutaneous placed tube (PTBD) draining bile points towards obstructive jaundice. Endoscopic biliary drainage (ENBD or biliary stent) is done for distal blocks (carcinoma HOP, periampullary cancer, distal cholangiocarcinoma) and is also preferred for proximal blocks when feasible, whereas PTBD is generally done for proximal blocks when endoscopically there is no access (for perihilar cholangiocarcinoma or GBC)
- *Past history*:
  - Past history of biliary stone disease—(typical epigastric pain radiating to infrascapular region, +/− fever/jaundice) gives a clue towards similar disease or GBC developing over a long period following repeated attacks of cholecystitis in genetically susceptible patients.
  - Past history of laparoscopic cholecystectomy could point towards the jaundice being secondary to BBS due to bile duct injury.
- *Family history predisposing to pancreatic cancer*:
  - Familial pancreatitis (Mutation in *PRSS1*, *SPINK1* and *CFTR* genes)
  - Familial adenomatosis polyposis (Germline mutation in *APC* gene)
  - Lynch syndrome (Germline mutation in mismatch repair genes)
  - Hereditary breast and ovarian cancer (Germline mutation in *BRCA* gene)

- *Performance history*: As per ECOG (Eastern Cooperative Oncology Group) classification to know if the patient will tolerate surgical stress or at least chemo/RT.

■ EXAMINATION PROFORMA

General Examination: Part A
- *Visual appearance*:
  - Young/middle aged/elderly
- *Gender*:
  - Male/female
- *Built*: Poor/average/good
- *Nourishment*: Poor/average/good
  - Measure height, weight, BMI

Clinical evaluation:
- Conscious/stuporous
- Cooperative/uncooperative
- Orientation to time, place and person: Present/absent
- Hydration status: Hydrated/dehydrated
- Lying comfortably bed/in discomfort/in pain
- Whether patient prefers sitting or lying down position
- Febrile/afebrile

Vitals: Pulse, BP, respiratory rate, mention performance status here as well

General Examination: Part B
- *Look for PICCLE, oral cavity, skin, features of CLD*:

PICCLE: Pallor, icterus, cyanosis, clubbing, generalized or localized lymphadeno-pathy, palpable cervical and left supraclavicular lymph node, pedal or dependent edema

Sites to look for icterus: Sclera/bulbar conjunctiva, undersurface of tongue, soft palate, palms and soles.

Examination of oral cavity: Look for oral hygiene and any obvious mucosal lesions, apart from jaundice.

Skin for scratch marks secondary to pruritus

Any stigmata of chronic liver disease (top to bottom):
  - Icterus
  - Malar erythema
  - Fetor hepaticus (thiols pass directly to lung)
  - Parotid swelling
  - Spider nevi/spider angiomata
  - Gynecomastia
  - Reduced chest hair
  - Reduced axillary hair
  - Dupuytren contracture

- Palmar erythema
- Leukonychia
- Flapping tremors/Asterixis
- Abdominal distension
- Caput medusae
- Reduced pubic hair
- Testicular atrophy
- Pedal edema

Abdominal Examination

Look for the presence of endoscopic nasobiliary drain (ENBD)/percutaneous transhepatic biliary drain (PTBD) as has been already discussed above.

On inspection See if:
- Abdominal contour: Flat/distended/scaphoid
- Umbilicus: Central/displaced. Inverted/everted/flat
- All quadrants are moving equally with respiration or not
- Any visible lump/nodule
- Distended gallbladder may be visible in right upper abdominal quadrant.

If visible describe:
- Size
- Site
- Shape
- Surface
- Movement with respiration

In a thin patient with bulky carcinoma HOP or GBC, a lump may be visible in mid upper abdomen, describe its:
- Site
- Size
- Shape
- Surface
- *Movement*: None with respiration.
- Look for visible scar (of previous laparoscopic cholecystectomy), sinus, engorged veins, pulsations, peristalsis or cough impulse.
- Inspect the groin hernial sites and examine genitalia.
- Inspection of renal angles to look for fullness

On palpation See if:
- Abdomen is soft, non-tender
- Liver is palpable or not (hepatomegaly may be present in case of liver metastasis)
- If palpable, measure its extent from costal margin in midclavicular line
- It is tender/nontender
- Consistency is soft/firm/hard
- Surface is smooth/nodular
- Borders are round/sharp, regular/irregular
- Margins

Gallbladder—palpable or not: As per Courvoisier's law: In OJ, a non-tender, palpable gallbladder is seldom due to gallstones (as the gallbladder is shrunken in chronic cholecystitis), exceptions being mucocele of the gallbladder due to stone obstructing the cystic duct and dual obstruction due to stones in CBD as well as gallbladder

Remember that generally gallbladder will be distended in distal blocks, but will be collapsed in proximal blocks:
- Spleen is enlarged or not
- Any other palpable lump as already discussed above

If present, then describe its:
- Site
- Size
- Shape
- Surface
- Margins
- Tenderness
- Consistency
- Mobility
- Movement with respiration
- *Plane*:
    - To help differentiate between abdominal wall and intra-abdominal masses, perform the leg raising test (also known as Carnett's test): a parietal mass will become more prominent while the patient raises their legs, while an intra-abdominal mass will become less prominent.
    - To help differentiate between intraperitoneal and retroperitoneal masses, perform the lateral decubitus test: A retroperitoneal mass will not fall ahead, while an intraperitoneal mass will.
- Palpate groin hernia sites and examine genitals
- Look for tenderness in renal angles
- Examine back and spine for tenderness.

On percussion:
- Look for upper border of liver dullness (generally in the 5th intercostal space) in midclavicular line.
- Note the liver span (normal being 12–14 cm)
- Percussion note over the gallbladder—dull note, continuous with that of liver dullness.
- Note the percussion note over rest of the abdomen
- Tests for free fluid. Presence of free fluid, i.e., ascites suggests metastatic disease in context of malignant obstructive jaundice.

On auscultation:
- Auscultate for bowel sounds.
- Bruit, hum and rub
- *Per-rectal examination*: Look for metastatic deposits in the pouch of Douglas (Blumer Shelf).

Respiratory examination

Rest systemic examination

■ CLINICAL DISCUSSION

Absence of prodromal symptoms, along with the presence of clay colored stools and dark urine, and a palpable gallbladder, all of these point toward surgical obstructive jaundice (SOJ) and not medical OJ (however, phase of intrahepatic cholestasis in medical OJ can also present with clay colored stools and dark urine, *but never with a palpable gallbladder*).

For painful progressive OJ, consider these two differentials:
1. *Head of pancreas cancer*:
   - Often associated with epigastric pain radiating to back, worsening with meals, relieved by bending forward, recent change in nature of pain in chronic pancreatitis (CP) (from intermittent to continuous dull aching).
   - Lump (palpable gallbladder or the mass itself) may be felt by the patient, may present with GOO and melena if it is infiltrating duodenum
   - Recent onset of diabetes in CP (within 2 years)/worsening of glycemic control, OR onset of diabetes after 50 years of age.
   - Associated with profound weight loss and loss of appetite as the presenting complaint most of the times.
2. *Gallbladder cancer*:
   - Associated with RHC pain (dull pain of liver infiltration and capsule stretch), and may be preceded by biliary colic/cholecystitis/cholangitis/pancreatitis due to stones.
   - May also be associated with GOO (though less often than HOP CA) and melena (if duodenal infiltration).

Whereas painless progressive OJ is seen with periampullary and perihilar cholangiocarcinoma (pHCC). However, after these two, we must always include HOP CA and GBC as well in the list, as it is not necessary to always have pain associated with these two.

Amongst malignant causes, periampullary cancer presents most commonly with cholangitis, followed by GBC also having stones or sludge. However remember that cholangitis is generally seen with benign diseases of biliary tree like stones, choledochal cyst (CDC), BBS, etc., and whereas the jaundice associated with stones, sludge and CDC is intermittent, a BBS presents generally with painless progressive jaundice.

Just remember that even if it is painless progressive jaundice, but there are some strong pointers like change in nature of pain in CP, or recent onset of diabetes mellitus (DM) in CP (within 2 years) or recent worsening of sugar control or onset after crossing 50, profound weight loss, then HOP CA must be considered the first diagnosis, followed by GBC, and then the other two. So clues like painless progressive jaundice are to be used only in context and these do not take precedence over other strong pointers.

Melena in malignant SOJ, can be seen in:
- Tumor of the papilla (due to sloughing, with waxing and waning jaundice)
- Duodenal periampullary (~25–30%)
- HOP CA infiltrating duodenum, and also if associated with CP, can cause splenic vein thrombosis and gastric varices, which may bleed.
- GBC infiltrating duodenum.

However, not having melena does not obviously rule out papillary or duodenal periampullary CA.

Just remember that gallbladder (even if it may be distended on USG) is palpable in only 50–60% of distal blocks. Also if there was chronic cholecystitis associated previously, then gallbladder would be contracted and hence would not be palpable. And lastly if patient underwent ERCP (endoscopic retrograde cholangiopancreatography) stenting for a distal block, even then gallbladder would not be palpable (except for GBC neck causing cystic duct block and mucocele).

Hence, even if gallbladder is not palpable, then along with pHCC, always still consider distal blocks in your differentials, especially if there are other pointers as well towards a gallbladder/pancreatic pathology. So if there is recent worsening of sugar control with painful progressive jaundice, and gallbladder is not palpable, HOP CA must be the first differential, followed by GBC (because it is painful progressive jaundice).

Also remember that, after ERCP/percutaneous transhepatic biliary drain (PTBD) stenting for malignant SOJ, if gallbladder is still palpable, that means either stent has not decompressed the system, or it is a GBC neck, and not a distal block, as stent will only decompress CBD (in which palpable gallbladder due to HOP CA/periampullary/distal cholangioca will collapse), but not cystic duct (which is blocked in GBC neck, leading to mucocele and distended palpable gallbladder).

CHAPTER 3.2

Hepatopancreatobiliary—Surgical Obstructive Jaundice Approach

■ APPROACH TO THE MANAGEMENT OF A HEPATOPANCREATOBILIARY CASE

First review all old records.
For all cases, say you want to review all previous investigations including:

Hemogram
Look for cytopenia, anemia-nutritional/bleed related, raised/low counts showing sepsis and low platelets representing hemolysis due to hypersplenism, and if <1 lakh, then even clinically significant pulmonary hypertension (PHTN) if there is associated gastrointestinal (GI) bleed or other signs.

Liver Function Tests (LFT)
Look for cholestasis, cholangitis, and especially for indicators of chronic liver disease (CLD) like high bilirubin, low albumin, albumin/globulin (A/G) reversal, and raised INR, and also calculate Child's score for CLD.

Remember that direct hyperbilirubinemia points to OJ, but indirect hyperbilirubinemia (IH) points toward hemolysis (in presence of splenomegaly due to any cause), cirrhosis [due to PHTN, splenomegaly causing hemolysis (correlate with increased reticulocyte count and peripheral blood film (PBF) showing target cells) and impaired conjugation due to liver dysfunction] and so always look for pigment gallstones and their associated complications in this case. IH can also be there due to Crigler–Najjar disease in absence of cirrhosis.

AG reversal can occur if there is low albumin due to malnutrition or poor liver synthetic function due to CLD/cirrhosis OR renal loss due to nephrotic syndrome OR AG reversal can occur if there is increased globulin production seen in infections, multiple myeloma, autoimmune diseases and cancers.

INR will be elevated in obstructed jaundice which will get corrected by vitamin K, and can even be deranged in sepsis.

Kidney Function Tests
High BUN points to dehydration, low urea points to liver dysfunction/CLD as urea is synthesized in the liver, and very low creatinine points to low muscle mass/catabolic state. eGFR based on age, sex, race, creatinine is important

as if it is <30 mL/min/m², then iodinated and gadolinium both contrasts are contraindicated.

Electrolytes

In cases with vomiting and/or diarrhea, as correction is required for the same before proceeding with further investigations.

Viral serology (routine workup) and USG abdomen pelvis, CXR, contrast-enhanced computed tomography (CECT), MR, upper gastrointestinal endoscopy (UGIE) any biopsy, ERCP any biopsy, and any previous operation records.

Then ask for two sets of investigations: (1) for diagnosis and staging, (2) another for workup-which includes routine blood investigations and special blood tests.

At the end of all investigations, do not forget to get cardiopulmonary evaluation (including ECG, 2D echo, PFT) *and optimization of patient* (nutrition, blood sugars, reviewing medication and physician and anesthesia consultation), *and MDT discussion* with detailed counseling before chemo/surgery with patient.

So for arriving at/confirming diagnosis and staging, *USG abdomen and CXR should be the first investigations always.* If CXR shows cannon ball metastases, then no further investigations are required and the intent of treatment becomes palliative. If USG abdomen suggests biliary stones/any cystic lesion/any pathology related to ducts, then first go for MRI with MRCP as the next investigation. If not, then can go ahead with CECT.

Criteria for IHBRD: Intrahepatic bile ducts (>2 mm or >40% of adjacent portal vein) and for extrahepatic (>6 +1 mm per decade above 60 years of age or >10 mm post-cholecystectomy).

Criteria for MPD dilatation: >3 mm in head and >2 mm in body and tail.

In case of a suspected periampullary pathology, if USG and CECT do not show any lesion, and CBD is dilated, but MPD is not dilated, that means lesion is most probably in distal CBD, so get an MRCP done, following which side-viewing endoscopy (SVE) with endoscopic ultrasound (EUS) and EUS guided biopsy OR ERCP and brush cytology/biopsy and can be done.

In case of a papillary type tumor within CBD, it is also better to get a complete spyglass cholangioscopy done as IPMNs can be multicentric.

If CBD and MPD both are dilated, and lesion is not seen on USG, CECT, then it may be a small periampullary papillary tumor, so still get an MRCP done first to localize the lesion, followed by SVE +– biopsy or EUS with guided biopsy or ERCP +– brush cytology/biopsy can be done.

Now when asking for fresh blood investigations, ask all the routine blood investigations as already listed above with the mentioned reasons (also amylase, lipase, calcium, lipid profile if needed for suspected pancreatitis) and viral serology.

Now only if USG shows anything specific, then ask for all other special blood tests.
- So if a solid liver lesion is seen, then ask for blood tests for diagnosing malignant lesions, as benign ones do not produce anything.

- So CEA (because metastases are commonest liver lesions), viral serology, AFP, PIVKA (for HCC), vitamin B12 binding globulin and neurotensin (for fibrolamellar HCC), CA19-9 (for cholangiocarcinoma), chromogranin A (for NET).
- And if cystic liver lesion seen, then based on history, ask for amoebic, hydatid serologies to rule out infective, then other tests to rule out noninfective (malignant ones only, as benign, premalignant and traumatic would not be produce anything), so CEA/CA-125 as metastases are most common, so cystic metastases from colorectal cancer (CRC)/ovarian CA, then viral serology, AFP, PIVKA for cystic HCC, chromogranin A for cystic NET and CA19-9 for BCAC (highly specific if above 600).

Blood CA19-9 Level:
It is sialated Lewis A blood group antigen (hence levels would not rise in patients who are Lewis antigen negative).

Levels rise in patients with pancreaticobiliary malignancies. It is however, not cancer specific and CA19-9 levels may rise in many benign HPB diseases (most importantly: Cholangitis). Hence levels are best performed after achieving biliary decompression, if they do not fall then consider malignancy.

Normal: < 37 U/mL

Role:
- Support diagnosis of pancreaticobiliary malignancies
- Assessing resectability (>1,000 likely metastatic)
- Assessing need for staging laparoscopy (indicated if levels are >100 U/mL as per NCCN)
- *Response assessment*: Postneoadjuvant therapy, postsurgery, postadjuvant therapy
- Surveillance

Remember that MRI with MRCP scores over CECT for cystic lesions of liver and pancreas (as it informs about cyst size/number/whether multifocal, wall thickness, mural nodules, internal septa, solid components, communication with ducts and dilatation) and to determine any ductal communication/anatomy/pathology like stones, strictures etc. Adding CE-MRI will also inform about intensity pattern of various lesions in arterial and portal venous (PV) phases, and also about vascular anatomy, signal voids, collaterals, etc.

MRI with MRCP also delineates longitudinal spread of cancer along ducts better, and should also be the first investigation in perihilar block. Adding MRA will complete the picture by highlighting vascular anatomy, relationship of lesion with vessels, signal voids signifying thrombosis as well as collaterals.

But keep in mind that CECT can also help in lesion characterization: CECT *shows radial spread better* even in perihilar cholangiocarcinoma, it is relationship with major vessels (better resolution than MRA), and *is definitely required for planning surgery* like CT volumetry for proximal lesions, *and is more preferred over MR for distal blocks, to assess the mass.*

Pancreatic adenocarcinoma appears hypoisodense in plain, hypoenhancing in late arterial aka pancreatic parenchymal phase and it's relationship with arteries is seen in this phase, then in portal venous phase it becomes isoenhancing and it's relationship is seen with SMV, PV and to assess liver metastases which look hypoenhancing to liver in this phase.

Whereas, NET is hyperenhancing in pancreatic parenchymal phase and even NET liver metastases are hyperenhancing in arterial and PV phases.

Contrast-enhanced computed tomography helps in deciding anatomical borderline resectability in pancreatic lesions and to assess vascular complications (pseudoaneurysm, thrombosis collaterals). CECT is required finally for staging to look for omental/pelvic deposits and other distant metastases.

And always say, you would like to discuss imaging with the radiologist also, before ordering a second investigation.

Whenever clinical situation demands (liver imaging atypical/inconclusive for NET, or atypical HCC or LIRADS not applicable as liver noncirrhotic or liver metastases with unknown primary—IHC needed to know organ of origin or BRPC), *get a biopsy done along with IHC.*

Get UGIE, SVE, EUS, ERCP, cholangioscopy, pancreatoscopy, and FNA/biopsy done whenever possible to complete workup and to get a definite diagnosis.

Also for complete staging, as per clinical situation: FDG PET CT/DOTATATE and even staging laparoscopy before laparotomy, and as far as possible try to get the diagnosis 100% beforehand by all possible safe means. Do not assume anything, don't be in a hurry to jump to anything, analyse all available data, and only then commit to a particular treatment.

In case the tumor is large, locally advanced, involving adjacent organs/vessels and patient needs prehabilitation, seriously consider having a tissue diagnosis with IHC, FDG PET/DOTA PET scan (whichever is applicable) followed by staging laparoscopy to completely stage the disease. Get cardiopulmonary evaluation done, counseling, then MDT discussion followed by NACT (3–4 cycles, to take care of micromets, to assess disease biology and downstage to improve R0 resection) followed by reassessment again with FDG PET and staging laparoscopy, followed finally with definitive surgery.

However, if in MDT it seems that patient would not be able to tolerate chemo/patient is in impending obstruction and may land up with bowel obstruction, etc., and if the lesion is resectable, then plan for upfront surgery.

Always do staging laparoscopy for complete staging before doing portal vein embolization (PVE) or starting chemo, reassessment after PVE and chemo, and finally before ANY definitive surgery.

3.3 CHAPTER

Hepatopancreatobiliary— Management of Cases besides Gallbladder Cancer

■ CYSTIC LESIONS OF PANCREAS

Diagnosis

For cystic lesions in head of pancreas especially for suspected intraductal papillary mucinous neoplasm (IPMN), *side-viewing endoscopy (SVE)* (showing fish mouth papilla with mucin oozing) and if possible, *EUS (endoscopic ultrasound) with cyst fluid analysis and pancreatoscopy and biopsy* of other synchronous intraductal lesions should be done.

Endoscopic ultrasound must be done in all cases of cystic lesions of pancreas, as it may show multicentric IPMN (seen in 20% cases), and for all cystic lesions, should report about cyst characteristics like size, wall thickness, septae, solid components, mural nodules, common bile duct (CBD), main pancreatic duct (MPD) dilatation, distal atrophy, nodal status, and also most importantly relationship of lesion with vessels Long contact with superior mesenteric vein (SMV) can preclude resection anastomosis.

Most importantly, EUS can characterize lesion by fine needle aspiration (FNA) and cyst fluid analysis. EUS FN core biopsy should be done in lesions in background of chronic pancreatitis (CP) to increase yield, as these lesions will have lot of fibrosis. Also to increase EUS biopsy yield, ROSE-Rapid on site evaluation can be done, so that if yield is poor, FNA can be repeated as scope is still inside.

Biochemical Analysis of Cyst Fluid (Table 1)

- Carcinoembryonic antigen (CEA) not predictive of malignancy, but accurate tumor marker for differentiating mucinous from non-mucinous pancreatic cysts[1]
- CEA does not distinguish IPMN from mucinous cystic neoplasm (MCN)
- CEA greater than 192 ng/mL: 73% sensitivity and 84% specificity for mucinous cysts[2]
- Cyst fluid glucose may be more accurate than CEA for mucinous cysts (recent meta-analysis: 91% sensitivity and 75% specificity for glucose compared with 67% sensitivity and 80% specificity for CEA)[3]

TABLE 1: Imaging paradigm of cystic lesions in pancreas (ILBS 2016).[8]

Fluid analysis of cystic pancreatic lesions						
Fluid characteristics	Pseudocyst	SCN	MCN	IPMN	SPN	CPEN
Cytology	No epithelium	Cuboidal epithelium	Columnar epithelium	Columnar epithelium	Branching papilla, myxoid stroma	Salt-and-pepper chromatin
Viscosity	Low	Low	High	High	Bloody fluid	Low
Mucin	Low	Low	Very High	Very High	NA	Low
CEA	Low	Low	High	High	NA	Low
CA 19-9	Low	Low	High	Variable	NA	Unknown
CA 72-4	Low	Low	High	High	NA	Unknown
Amylase	Very High	Low	Variable	High	NA	Low
Glycogen	Absent	Very high	Absent	Absent	NA	Absent
DNA KRAS	Absent	Absent	Present	Present	Unknown	Unknown

(CPEN: cystic pancreatic endocrine neoplasm; IPMN: intraductal-papillary mucinous neoplasm; KRAS: Kirsten rat sarcoma viral oncogene homolog; MCN: mucinous cystic neoplasm; NA: not applicable; SCN: serous cystic neoplasm; SPN: solid pseudopapillary neoplasm)

- Cutoff commonly used for cyst fluid glucose in diagnosing mucinous cysts is <50 mg/dL
- Very low CEA levels <5 ng/mL: Specific for serous cystadenoma (SCA), pseudocyst, or cystic neuroendocrine tumor[4]
- Amylase <250 U/L: Pseudocyst excluded[4]

DNA Analysis of Cyst Fluid

- Done when <0.5 mL fluid available (such less volume not amenable to biochemical tests)
- KRAS (Kirsten rat sarcoma viral oncogene homolog) and GNAS (guanine nucleotide binding protein, alpha stimulating) mutations more accurate for diagnosing mucinous cysts and IPMNs than CEA alone (recent meta-analysis)[5] GNAS is specific for IPMN
- Some preliminary studies of various DNA mutation panels suggest high sensitivity and specificity for identifying cysts with high-grade dysplasia or cancer[6,7]

Remember that SCN, MCN, solid pseudopapillary neoplasm (SPEN) are focal lesions, whereas IPMN can have multiple diffusely spread lesions along with a dilated main pancreatic duct (MPD). In around 10% even MCN can communicate with MPD.

Multiple cystic lesions in pancreas can also be as a part of autosomal dominant polycystic kidney disease (ADPKD) with renal and liver cysts, also acinar cell neoplasm can look like that (spongy pancreas).

CHAPTER 3.3: Hepatopancreatobiliary—Management of Cases besides Gallbladder Cancer

Surgical Resection

- Surgical resection is recommended for symptomatic serous cystic neoplasms (SCNs) only[9,10]
- Resection of MCNs should be considered for all patients or select higher risk patients with symptoms, nodule or size ≥ 4 cm[10,11]
- Surgical resection is suggested for main-duct intraductal papillary mucinous neoplasm (MD-IPMN) and mixed type IPMNs due to higher malignant risk[10,11]
- *Absolute indications for resection of Branch-duct IPMN (BD-IPMN)*: Main pancreatic duct ≥ 1 cm, jaundice, enhancing nodule ≥ 5 mm, solid mass, or cytology suspicious or positive for malignancy.
- *Relative indications for resection of BD-IPMN*: Main pancreatic duct 5–9 mm, cyst ≥ 4 cm, enhancing nodule < 5 mm, growth rate ≥ 5 mm/year, serum CA 19-9 ≥ 37 U/mL, acute pancreatitis, or new onset diabetes.
- *SPENs*: Premalignant; ~15% incidence of local invasion or metastatic disease.[12] Occurrence mainly in young women, with favorable post-resection outcomes, hence surgical resection preferred.[9,10]
- MD-IPMN with segmental dilation or diffuse dilation with focal lesions: Partial pancreatectomy advised[11]
- *MD-IPMN with diffuse dilation without focal lesions*: Total pancreatectomy in young (Can tolerate brittle diabetes and exocrine insufficiency) versus all patients with diffuse main pancreatic duct dilation or those with family history of pancreatic cancer[10,11]

In resections for cystic lesions, consent must be taken for major resection, including total pancreatosplenectomy.

Intraoperative pancreatoscopy must be done and margin must always be sent for frozen as IPMN is a field defect, so there may be multicentric lesions, and also IPMN is sentinel for pancreatic cancer, so there can also be synchronous cancer.

If more lesions seen via scopy, or high-grade dysplasia (HGD)/malignancy at margin, then further resection must be done and again confirmed with frozen, and if duct is diffusely dilated with multiple lesions, consider total pancreatosplenectomy, which is however morbid due to brittle diabetes (recurrent episodes of hypoglycemia as even glucagon is lost).

Surveillance

- *MRI preferred over CT*: Reduced radiation exposure and improved ability to detect communication with the main pancreatic duct and nodules[9,10,13]
- *Non-contrast MRI*: Similar efficacy to contrast-enhanced MRI in discerning benign from malignant disease[14]
- *Post-surgical resection of SCN or MCN without invasive features*: Surveillance not necessary as resection curative (No recurrence of MCN without invasive cancer after nearly 5 years)[15]
- *Higher risk IPMNs including high-grade dysplasia at the surgical margins, non-intestinal subtype, or family history of pancreatic cancer, Fukuoka guideline*: Repeat imaging at least every 6 months.[11]

- *For other IPMNs*, surveillance every 6–12 months is suggested.
- *Resected invasive cancer*: Surveillance as per patients with pancreatic ductal adenocarcinoma

All efforts must be made to get a preoperative diagnosis/biopsy without increasing chances of metastatic spread due to it. So for hepatobiliary lesions either EUS guided biopsy, or ERCP with brush cytology, or spyglass endoscopic/cholangioscopic biopsy or even percutaneous transhepatic cholangiography (PTC) and biopsy for indeterminate high intrahepatic strictures and for pancreas: EUS guided biopsy or pancreatoscopy and biopsy, etc., must be done.

Also, FDG PET CT and staging laparoscopy must be done before all major hepatopancreatobiliary (HPB) resections especially like extended right hepatectomy (ERH), hepatopancreatoduodenectomy (HPD)—for gallbladder cancer (GBC) or cholangiocarcinoma with above and downward spread, also in poorly differentiated hepatocellular carcinoma (HCC) with alpha-fetoprotein (AFP) >400, or before transplant with extended criteria, also locally advanced/borderline pancreatic cancer, pancreatic body/tail cancer, large nodes seen on CECT or when CA 19-9 is above 100. For such a pancreatic lesion, FDG PET CT changes management in ~20%.

■ HEAD OF PANCREAS CANCER (HOP CA)

Routine biliary drainage is not recommended for distal blocks. It is better done selectively (DROP trial).

Indications:
- Uncontrolled cholangitis (i.e., not responding to intensive medical management with IV antibiotics)
- Severe pruritus affecting the quality of life and sanity
- Coagulopathy
- Renal insufficiency
- Poor nutritional status/patient requires prehabilitation
- When neoadjuvant therapy is being planned in resectable or borderline resectable disease
- Surgery delayed due to any other reason
- When palliation is to be achieved in unresectable disease

Resectable Pancreas Cancer—Management
- *Upfront surgery followed by adjuvant chemo*
- *Head of pancreas cancer*: WHIPPLE [pylorus-preserving pancreaticoduodenectomy (PPPD)/pylorus-resecting pancreaticoduodenectomy (PRPD)]
- *CA Body/Tail*: Radical antegrade modular pancreatosplenectomy (RAMPS) (anterior/posterior—depending upon location of tumor with respect to posterior pancreatic capsule)

Borderline Resectable Pancreatic Cancer (BRPC)

Three different types of borderline resectable pancreatic ductal adenocarcinoma (BR-PDAC) (1) BR-type A: Anatomic features—relationship between the tumor and peripancreatic vessels; (2) BR-type B: Biological factors that raise the possibility (but not certainty) of extra-pancreatic metastatic disease; and (3) BR-type C: Conditional criteria, such as the performance status and patient comorbidities, which significantly increase the risk for morbidity or mortality after surgery.

National Comprehensive Cancer Network (NCCN) 2021 Anatomical Criteria for BRPC

Pancreatic Head/Uncinate Process Cancer

Arterial

Superior mesenteric artery (SMA): Solid tumor contact ≤ 180°; common hepatic artery (CHA): Solid tumor contact without extension to celiac artery (CA) or hepatic artery bifurcation allowing for safe and complete resection and reconstruction; Solid tumor contact with variant arterial anatomy (e.g., accessory right hepatic artery, replaced right hepatic artery, replaced CHA, and the origin of replaced or accessory artery).

Pancreatic Body/Tail Cancer

Arterial

Solid tumor contact < 180°; CA: Solid tumor contact ≥180° without involvement of the aorta and with intact and uninvolved gastroduodenal artery thereby permitting a modified Appleby procedure.

Venous (For Pancreatic Head /Uncinate Process Cancer as well as Pancreatic Body/Tail Cancer)

Superior mesenteric vein/portal vein (PV): Solid tumor contact ≥180°, contact of < 180° with contour irregularity of the vein or thrombosis of the vein but with suitable vessel proximal and distal to the site of involvement allowing for safe and complete resection and vein reconstruction.

Inferior vena cava (IVC): Solid tumor contact.

International association of pancreatology (IAP) consensus definition for BR-type B: "Tumor potentially resectable anatomically with clinical findings suspicious for, but not proven distant metastasis, including CA 19-9 level more than 500 units/mL, or regional lymph nodes metastasis diagnosed by biopsy or PET/CT".

IAP consensus definition for BR-type C: "Patients with anatomically resectable PDAC and with performance status of two or more".

For BRPC disease/any large distant nodes seen, EUS guided biopsy of lesion/nodes must be done. After confirming cancer by biopsy and after MDT discussion, NACT with mFOLFIRINOX or Gemcitabine and nab-paclitaxel or GemCap is given to downstage and see tumor biology (Days 1, 8 followed by 14 day gap and then Day 21) following which FDG PET CT/CECT have to be repeated before definitive surgery.

For BRPC body/tail modified Appleby, i.e., distal pancreatectomy with celiac axis resection (DP-CAR) can be done. Before that, CHA may be ligated to increase collateral flow from SMA via gastroduodenal artery (GDA) to the liver. In this waiting period, NACT is administered and response is assessed

■ PANCREATIC NEUROENDOCRINE TUMOR (PNET)

Diagnosis
- If CECT shows a hyperenhancing lesion in the pancreatic parenchymal (delayed arterial phase), then the lesion is most likely to be a neuroendocrine tumor.
- Biopsy must be done to know the differentiation (well or poorly) and grade (based on mitotic rate and Ki-67 proliferative index) as per latest WHO classification **(Table 2)**.

Immunohistochemical examination of the tumor to be done:
- General NET markers→chromogranin and synaptophysin
- Markers for the site of origin for neuroendocrine liver metastases (NELM) of unknown origin. PAX6, PAX8 and ISL1→pancreatic markers, CDX2 → small bowel NET and TTF1 → lung NET.
- Serum chromogranin A (CgA) → disease burden and survival.[17]
- Falsely elevated in hypertension, renal dysfunction and treatment with proton-pump inhibitors
- PCR-based assay (NETest) has recently been developed for the diagnosis and surveillance of NETs. Superior sensitivity and specificity (94% and 96%, respectively) for PNETs when compared to CgA; however more expensive[18]

TABLE 2: WHO 2019 classification of GEP-NEN.[16]

Terminology	Differentiation	Grade	Mitotic rate[a]	Ki-67 index[b]
NET, G1	Well-differentiated	Low	<2	<3%
NET, G2		Intermediate	2–20	3–20%
NET, G3		High	>20	>20%
SCNEC	Poorly differentiated	High	>20	>20%
LCNEC		High	>20	>20%
MiNEN	Well or poorly differentiated	Variable	Variable	Variable

[a]Mitotic rate: The number of mitoses per 2 mm^2.
[b]Ki-67 index: Counting ≥500 cells in the regions of highest labeling (hot-spots) which are identified at scanning magnification.
(LCNEC: large cell neuroendocrine carcinoma; MiNEN: mixed neuroendocrine non-neuroendocrine neoplasm; NEC: neuroendocrine carcinoma; NENs: neuroendocrine neoplasms; NET: neuroendocrine tumor; SCNEC: small cell neuroendocrine carcinoma)
Source: Klimstra DS, Kloppel G, La Rosa S, Rindi G. Digestive System Tumors. In: WHO Classification of Tumors. 5th edition. Vol 1. IARC, Lyon, 2019.

Insulinomas characterized by Whipple's triad: Hypoglycemic symptoms, low plasma glucose, and resolution of symptoms with administration of glucose. The diagnosis should be confirmed by measurement of elevated insulin, pro-insulin and C-peptide during a hypoglycemic episode, induced by a supervised 72-hour fast. In patients with refractory peptic ulcer disease, the presence of a gastrinoma may be confirmed by serum gastrin >10 times the upper limit of normal in the setting of gastric pH ≤ 2, or moderately elevated gastrin with a positive secretin or glucagon stimulation test. Proton-pump inhibitors should be discontinued for 2 weeks prior to measurement of the fasting serum gastrin, during which time acid suppression may be maintained with histamine type 2 blockers.

- Somatostatin receptors are expressed by 80–100% of PNETs, with the exception of insulinomas for which the rate of expression is 50–70%.[19]
- 68Ga-PET: Highest sensitivity (93%) and specificity (91%) for the diagnosis of NETs.[20]
- FDG-PET→for imaging poorly differentiated tumors, as they are less likely to express somatostatin receptors, and thus less likely to light up on 68Ga-PET.
- EUS→most sensitive test for localizing small PNETs, and also allows for biopsy to confirm the diagnosis.[21]

Management

Multidisciplinary→surgery, somatostatin analogs (SSAs), targeted therapy, and cytotoxic chemotherapy.

Surgery is the mainstay of treatment for PNETs[22] and is curative for localized disease. Even those with distant metastases derive significant benefit in terms of both symptom control and survival from surgical debulking.[23]

Localized Disease

- All PNETs >2 cm and functional tumors, irrespective of size, should be resected.[22]
- Reviews of the SEER and NCDB databases → Nearly 30% of PNETs <2 cm had nodal involvement, and thus malignant potential
- Studies supporting the safety of observation had relatively short follow-up. A meta-analysis comparing resection to nonsurgical management found that surgery was associated with a significant overall survival benefit, even for PNETs < 2 cm.[24]
- Enucleation can be considered for tumors which are well-circumscribed, small, well-differentiated, not in close proximity to the pancreatic duct, and without evidence of nodal or distant metastases.[25]
- Advantage of enucleation over standard pancreatic resection→lower rate of postoperative pancreatic insufficiency.[26]
- Disadvantage of enucleation → higher rate of postoperative pancreatic fistula.[27]
- Small tumors in the pancreatic body too close to the duct for safe enucleation may be resected via central pancreatectomy.[26]
- Formal pancreatic resection → for tumors >2 cm, abutting the pancreatic duct, intermediate or high grade, or suspicious for lymph node involvement.[26]

- Pancreaticoduodenectomy is performed for tumors of the pancreatic head, while tumors in the body or tail are resected via distal pancreatectomy, with or without splenic preservation. Regional lymphadenectomy should be performed with pancreatic resection, >50% of tumors >2 cm will have nodal metastases. Recurrence seen even after R0 resection, and more likely in disease with nodal metastases.[28]
- Surveillance with CT or MRI and CgA.
- Follow-up initially at 3–6 months, and then every 6–12 months and more frequent for high-grade tumors.
- Surveillance should be continued for at least 7 years following resection as late recurrences are seen. ^{68}Ga-PET is used to evaluate equivocal evidence of disease recurrence.[29]

Metastatic Disease

- Surgery plays a central role.[25]
- The liver accounts for about 80% of all metastases from pNETs, but metastases to the bone, distant lymph nodes, and peritoneal cavity (by direct invasion) are also frequent.[30]
- Among patients with metastatic disease, liver failure is the most common cause of death.
- Recent studies have shown improved survival and symptomatic control even with 70% debulking.

Criteria for debulking:
- Well-differentiated, grade 1 or 2, metastatic PNETs with <50% hepatic replacement with a surgically amenable distribution (i.e., not miliary), normal or near-normal liver function, and no evidence of carcinoid heart disease or other major comorbidities. Extrahepatic metastases should not be considered a contraindication to hepatic debulking, and peritoneal tumor deposits may be resected concurrently.[23]
- For patients with extensive liver involvement who are ineligible for hepatic debulking, but are otherwise well-suited for surgery and have no evidence of extrahepatic disease, liver transplantation appears to offer improved survival.[31]
- The indications for transplant, as defined by the Milan-NET criteria are very similar to those for hepatic debulking, further complicating patient selection.
- Primary tumor resection should be considered in patients with metastatic disease to avoid obstructive complications from the pancreatic mass and further metastatic seeding. In most cases this may be performed simultaneously; the primary exception is for pancreaticoduodenectomy and hepatic ablation, which should be performed in a staged manner to avoid risk of hepatic abscess formation. Even in the case of unresectable metastatic disease, there may be a survival advantage associated with resection of the primary tumor.[32]
- Primary tumor resection in the presence of unresectable liver metastases may be beneficial for functioning neoplasms to ameliorate symptoms and those with non functional (NF)-pancreatic NET (PanNET) G1–G2 located in the pancreatic body/tail with a good performance status.

- Surgery with radical intent may represent a valuable option for patients with PanNET-G3 and it may be considered even in the presence of metastatic disease. In contrast, surgery for localized pancreatic NEC (neuroendocrine carcinoma)-G3 should be considered with extreme caution, whereas it should be completely avoided in case of M+ PanNEC-G3.[33]

Management VHL and MEN1 Associated pNET

Tumors >3 cm in size, with doubling time <500 days, or exon 3 mutations are more likely to metastasize, and thus are indications for resection in VHL patients.[34]

Around 30–80% of patients diagnosed with MEN1 develop NF-PanNET. Surgical resection is recommended for patients with neoplasms ≥2 cm. In contrast, a surveillance management is usually offered to MEN1 patients with small lesions.[35,36]

Liver Directed Therapy

- Percutaneous ablation of liver metastases may be performed using radio-frequency ablation (RFA), microwave ablation (MWA), or cryoablation.
- Hepatic artery embolization (HAE) is indicated for patients with liver dominant disease and a patent portal vein who are not candidates for operative hepatic debulking.[25]
- Bland HAE is performed using polyvinyl alcohol particles which occlude blood flow to the metastases, inducing hypoxic necrosis. Chemotherapy or radioactive microspheres may also be delivered via the catheter, (chemoembolization and radioembolization, respectively).[37]
- Patients are admitted following embolization for the management of post-embolization syndrome. This self-limited syndrome is characterized by fever, abdominal pain, nausea and vomiting and occurs in up to 90% of patients following the procedure.[38]

Medical Therapy

- Long-acting somatostatin analogs (SSAs) are considered first line therapy for metastatic PNETs.[25]
- The tyrosine kinase inhibitor sunitinib and the mTOR inhibitor everolimus are second line and are associated with modest improvements in progression-free survival.[39,40]
- Capecitabine–Temozolomide (CAPTEM) has been introduced as a promising new regimen with high objective response rates, improved survival and superior tolerability.[41]
- Peptide receptor radionuclide therapy (PRRT) was shown to significantly increase progression-free survival (PFS) in patients with metastatic NETs in the NETTER trials. PRRT was recently FDA approved for the treatment of all NETs.[42]
- Standard first line chemotherapy for high-grade PNETs consists of cisplatin or carboplatin plus etoposide or irinotecan.[43]

PERIHILAR CHOLANGIOCARCINOMA (PHCC)

For pHCC, when planning hepatectomy, always try to get a preoperative tissue diagnosis with cholangioscopy and if right hepatectomy or extended right hepatectomy (ERH) planned and then do preoperative biliary drainage (PBD) of future liver remnant (FLR) segments to bring bilirubin below 3 before surgery (takes 2-3 weeks). Endoscopic methods especially endoscopic nasobiliary drainage (ENBD) and endoscopic biliary drainage (EBD) preferred over percutaneous transhepatic biliary drainage (PTBD) as PTBD has increased risk of tumor seeding, bleeding and bile leak as shown by Japanese Nagoya group.

Biliary Drainage Options in Proximal Blocks

- *ENBD* does not entail a sphincterotomy, hence reflux of pancreato-enteric contents does not occur in the biliary system, and hence does not predispose to cholangitis and biliary strictures. Also, it can be used for imaging the biliary system and bile refeeding can be done if bile is clear and culture is negative. Hence, it is currently the preferred method of biliary decompression
- *ERCP and EBD with stent*: Violates the sphincter and hence reflux of pancreato-enteric contents may occur in the biliary system which predisposes to cholangitis and biliary strictures.
- *PTBD*: As discussed above, may lead to biliary leak and bleeding (and also dissemination of malignancy if done for proximal blocks especially pHCC), hence least preferred technique. Was previously the workhorse in high volume Japanese Centers (Nagoya) but the above cited reasons have led to Japanese surgeons preferring ENBD and EBD whenever feasible, over PTBD.

Surgical Management

For types 1/2/3a lesion we do classical right hepatectomy with caudate resection [and left hepatic duct (LHD) margin is sent for frozen] along with extrahepatic bile duct resection [and lower end of CBD sent for frozen, if +, pancreaticoduodenectomy (PD) needs to be done] and all lymph node (LN) retrieval to the right of celiac, but if middle hepatic artery (MHA) is involved, then we may need to do extended right hepatectomy (ERH) as sacrificing MHA generally causes segment 4 ischemia, though at times MHA can be sacrificed without causing ischemia and then segment 4 may be preserved.

For type 3b lesion we do classical left hepatectomy with caudate resection [and right hepatic duct (RHD) margin is sent for frozen], along with extrahepatic bile duct resection (and lower end of CBD sent for frozen, if +, do PD) and all LN retrieval to the right of celiac.

For type 4 lesion it depends which side the tumor involvement is more, accordingly ERH or extended left hepatectomy (ELH) is done, along with extrahepatic bile duct resection (and lower end of CBD sent for frozen, if present, do PD) and all LN retrieval to the right of celiac. ELH, in other words—left trisectionectomy is preferred as right posterior section has good volume and hence FLR is good.

Thus, if ERH/ELH is planned (type 4 bismuth) and if FLR is inadequate, then after preoperative biliary drainage (PBD) once bilirubin <3, first do staging laparoscopy. If deposits are present, confirm with frozen and if metastatic, then refer for palliative chemo (even giving chemo requires bilirubin to be normalized). If no deposits, then do portal vein embolization (PVE) of tumor side segments and repeat CT volumetry after 3 weeks and staging laparoscopy immediately before surgery.

There is a French multicentre trial for PBD for right versus left hepatectomy for pHCC, so for right, PBD is beneficial, but for left it is detrimental (more infections and morbidity, less benefit).

Extended resections in pHCC as per Nagino are of two types:
1. Hepatopancreatoduodenectomy (HPD)
2. Portal vein/arterial resection-reconstruction

Super extended resection is defined as combination of both. It has high morbidity, but 5-year OS of up to 25–30% can be achieved.

Mayo criteria: Good candidates for liver transplantation for pHCC have "solitary, less than 3 cm in diameter, no lymph node metastases but unresectable tumor."

But as per Masato Nagino: Most pHCC meeting the Mayo criteria are not unresectable, but resectable. Extended resections, including trisectionectomy, HPD, vascular resections, can circumvent unnecessary transplantation and offer a favorable outcome even in locally advanced pHCC. However, those with primary sclerosing cholangitis (PSC) developing pHCC are good candidates for liver transplantation.

Benign lesion resembling pHCC: Post bile duct injury (BDI) benign biliary stricture (BBS), PSC, primary biliary cirrhosis (PBC), TB, IgG4 disease. However, presence of mass makes pHCC more likely.

HEPATOCELLULAR CARCINOMA

Diagnosis

For suspected HCC, CXR to rule out obvious cannon ball metastasis and USG abdomen with Doppler [To see liver echotexture, intrahepatic biliary radicle dilatation (IHBRD), space occupying lesion (SOL) characterization whether solid or cystic, relationship with vessels, PV thrombosis and collaterals, LN, omental/pelvic deposits and ascites and spleen].

Then blood tests: Bilirubin [1.1–1.9: limited resection only. ≥2: No resection, and the available options are: Transplant or Ablation or transarterial chemoembolisation (TACE)/transarterial radioembolisation (TARE)/systemic chemo] with viral serology, AFP (> 400, HCC diagnosis is >95% confirmed, and ≥1,000, transplant is contraindicated, post-TACE/TARE if it comes <500, transplant can be reconsidered), PIVKA, CEA, CA 19-9. Do serum vitamin B12 binding globulin and neurotensin for fibrolamellar HCC (FHCC) if suspected.

UGIE to look for varices [Presence of varices signifies portal hypertension (PHTN)+, then no resection to be done, and the available options are Transplant or Ablation or TACE/TARE/systemic chemo].

Liver protocol CECT chest, abdomen, pelvis to see lung metastasis, pleural effusion, liver surface whether nodular, irregular, lesion characterization, any PV thrombosis making it STAGE C BCLC, any LN (poor prognostic factor), metastatic deposits, ascites.

Bone Scan and FDG PET CT

If *AFP* >400, lesion is poorly differentiated, ERH is planned or Transplant with extended criteria.

Staging and Management

Stage as per BCLC: As per anatomical concerns: Size, no. of lesions, *biological concerns*: AFP, liver status by child's/ALBI score, PHTN *and conditional*: Comorbidities, performance status (PS) by ECOG score, six minute walk test (6MWT), stair climbing. If deranged bilirubin and portal hypertension are present then plan for transplant/ablation. In the absence of above, plan resection. If not fit enough due to non-liver factors or conditional concerns, then it automatically becomes stage D and needs best supportive care.

Before surgery do CT volumetry. FLR = (FLR volume/Tumor free liver volume) × 100. *Along with functional assessment* with Child's score, model for end-stage liver disease (MELD), hyder risk score: Clavien Dindo+ creatinine, bilirubin, INR (CBI), *ALBI, EZ-ALBI and APRI scores, ICG retention—**Makuuchi criteria based on ascites, bilirubin, ICG and then finally hepatobiliary (HB) scintigraphy: Tc99m GSA or mebrofenin/HIDA (least affected by bilirubin levels and allows

---

* *ALBI*: Logarithmic score based on albumin and bilirubin with 3 grades (1-best, 3-worst), and a refined version of Child's score. Detection of the small changes in liver function in compensated cirrhosis that the Child and MELD are not sensitive enough to detect. Strongly associated with the degree of hepatic fibrosis, as assessed by the *FIB-4* (fibrosis-4) index or aspartate aminotransferase-to-platelet ratio index (APRI).

The best documented risk score for HCC in patients with CLD is the *aMAP score* which combines ALBI with male sex, age and platelets.

$$EZ\text{-}ALBI: [T.Bil\ (mg/dL)] - [9 \times Alb\ (g/dL)]$$

this value highly correlated with the ALBI score.

APRI: Determines the likelihood of hepatic fibrosis and cirrhosis in Hepatitis C.

** *Makuuchi criteria*: If ascites uncontrolled, and/or bilirubin is ≥2, then no need to do ICG, and no resection to be done.

If ascites is controlled and bilirubin 1.1–1.9, then again, no need to do ICG, and only limited resection to be done.

Only if no/controlled ascites, and bilirubin is ≤1, then ICG—Retention at 15 minutes to be done:
- ICG <10%: Trisectionectomy
- 10–19%: RH/LH
- 20–29%: Subsegmentectomy
- 30% and above: Limited resection.

regional function and thus FLR assessment) combined with SPECT, *and plan for PVE if needed* (after staging laparoscopy).

Repeat CT volumetry after 3 weeks of PVE: Degree of hypertrophy >5% has better outcomes, repeat functional assessment. HB scintigraphy for FLR function—<2.69%/min/m² uptake and also ICG plasma disappearance rate <17.6% is associated with high rates of posthepatectomy liver failure (PHLF) and also do staging laparoscopy just before surgery.

Latest BCLC Stage B allows transplant beyond Milan as per UCSF/other extended criteria, also if TACE and TARE (for those beyond extended) can downstage to within extended criteria, transplant can be done.

BCLC Stage C involves palliative chemo only with first line being atezolizumab (PD-L1 inhibitor) + bevacizumab, based on the IMBrave150 trial comparing with sorafenib, so atezo-bev showed OS of 19 months versus 10–13 months with sorafenib. Recent meta-analysis has shown atezo-bev to be safe even in Child–Turcotte–Pugh (CTP) B score.

However, varices must be obliterated before their use, otherwise they can precipitate bleeding diathesis. So in such a case with high grade varices not obliterated, Tyrosine kinase inhibitors (TKIs) like sorafenib or lenvatinib or regorafenib or cabozantinib, and even TARE should be used.

Now BCLC simplified for HCC:
- So if PS 1–2/PV invasion/extrahepatic disease, it becomes Stage C
- And if PS 3–4 OR end-stage liver, it becomes Stage D
- Rest all stages include PS 0 and preserved liver function

Resection is the option only for a single lesion:
- So if ≤2 cm it's stage 0, and if not a candidate for transplant, then ablation. And if a candidate, then see bilirubin and portal pressure. So if bilirubin and portal pressure normal, then resection to be done. If bilirubin and portal pressure raised, then see if any contraindication for transplant. If yes, then ablation. If no, then transplant.
- And if size >2 cm, upto any size, then it's Stage A. As you've to resect, again see bilirubin and portal pressure and do as above. (Remember even if bilirubin and portal pressure raised, then resection can still be done for a peripheral HCC).

Now if >1 lesion, then no resection:
- 3 lesions and up to 3 cm each is Stage A.
- >3 lesions/>3 cm each is Stage B.

So the options available are:
- Transplant (Milan for stage A/Extended criteria for Stage B)
- Ablation (if any contraindication for transplant) OR
- TACE for Stage B—well defined nodules with preserved portal flow and those even out of extended criteria for transplant OR for any lesions in which ablation/resection/transplant cannot be done OR
- TARE (in those with portal flow issues, *only for single lesion ≤ 8 cm*).

Diffuse bilateral involvement of Stage B OR

Advanced Stage C (PS 1-2 OR PV thrombosis OR extrahepatic spread) OR

When TACE/TARE are not feasible, the only option is systemic treatment.

In systemic treatment:
- *1st line*: Atezo-bev/Durvalumab-tremelimumab
  if not feasible, then Sorafenib/Lenvatinib
- *2nd line after sorafenib*: Regorafenib/Ramucirumab (for AFP ≥400)
- *3rd line*: Cabozantinib
  If all these given/post-atezo-bev/post-Durvalumab-tremelimumab/not feasible, enrol in trials.

Stage D (PS 3-4, end-stage liver disease): Best supportive care (BSC)

NEUROENDOCRINE LIVER METASTASIS (NELM)

NELM patterns:
- *Type 1*: Restricted to one lobe or 2 adjacent segments. Can be anatomically resected.
- *Type 2*: One dominant lesion (resectable) with satellite nodules in contralateral side which need ablation or two-staged resection
- *Type 3*: Diffuse, multifocal. Debulking, transplant and chemo are options.

Liver transplant criteria in NELM:

MILAN: (Mazzaferro: 5-year OS 90%)
- Well differentiated G1/G2 liver NET
- <50% liver involvement
- Liver NET stable/responsive ≥6 months prior to transplant
- Primary drained by portal system and removed
- Age <60 (relative)

ENETS: Additionally, absence of extra hepatic disease (which is obvious) and postoperative mortality to be <10%.

Systemic chemo for metastatic unresponsive G3 NETs and all NECs:
As per NORDIC registry, for Grade 3 NENs
- Ki67 <55: CAPTEM
- Ki67 >55: Etoposide/platinum

A SMALL NOTE ON LIVER RESECTION

Types of vascular control:
- Total vascular inflow control (Pringle)
- Selective (Hemi, sectional, segmental)
- Total Hepatic Vascular Exclusion (with or without preservation of caval flow)
- Selective

Approaches:
- *Intrafascial*: Traditional hilar dissection (extrahepatic). Can also be done intrahepatically. Hilar structures are dissected individually within the sheath. Dangerous, can damage structures of FLR.

- *Extrafascial*:
  - Extrahepatic (Suprahilar glissonean pedicle approach)
  - Intrahepatic (Transfissural anterior/posterior), posterior eliminates disadvantages of intrafascial as well as extrafascial.

It is safe as individual structures not dissected separately, but taken en masse as they all lie within the glissonean pedicle. Can be used to perform any anatomical resection safely.

Approaches to right hepatectomy:
- *Conventional approach*: Ligation of caudate veins draining into IVC and few from portal vein, Inflow control, liver mobilization (dissection of coronary and triangular ligaments) ligation of all short hepatic veins, outflow control with ligation of right hepatic vein and then finally parenchymal transection.
- *Anterior approach (done for massive tumors that may cause rupture, avulsion of veins, ischemic damage to FLR due to rotation done for control of outflow during conventional approach)*: Ligation of caudate veins draining into IVC and few from portal vein, Inflow control, Liver hanging maneuver (Belghiti), parenchymal transection, followed by ligation of all short hepatic veins and then finally control and ligation of hepatic vein, followed by liver mobilization (dissection of coronary and triangular ligaments) and extraction of specimen.

OTHER BENIGN DISEASES

■ ORIENTAL CHOLANGIOHEPATITIS (OCH)

Saharia criteria for primary CBD stones:
- >2 years since Cholecystectomy
- No long cystic duct remnant
- Soft brown Earthy stones

So first USG abdomen to look for liver echotexture, any space occupying lesion (SOL), any filling defects in ducts, IHBRD, stones in CHD, GB, CBD, size of CBD, lymphadenopathy. Also to look for portal vein thrombosis (PVT), collaterals, ascites, Splenomegaly—signs of secondary biliary cirrhosis (SBC) with portal hypertension (PHTN) due to recurrent episodes of cholangitis.

Then ask for MRI with MRCP, to look for:
- Liver surface (smooth/can be nodular in long-standing cases signifying CLD, SBC), any crowding of ducts signifying atrophy hypertrophy complex (AHC), extent of liver whether extending up to spleen, any cholangiolytic abscesses, ductal anatomy, any signal voids inside, any dominant strictures, any signal voids in CHD, GB, CBD.
- *Look for any suspicious mass lesion* (OCH predisposes to cholangiocarcinoma). Also for disproportionate dilatation that maybe a choledochal cyst (CDC), then look at lower end smooth tapering/stricture, main pancreatic duct (MPD) and if any anomalous pancreaticobiliary ductal junction (APBDJ) (union outside duodenal wall or ≥15 mm).
- Also look for splenomegaly.

Now *MR angiogram (MRA) may be done for vascular anatomy or ask for CECT* to look for vascular anatomy, PVT, venous collaterals, splenomegaly.
- *If any signs of SBC, then do fibroscan to grade fibrosis/cirrhosis and UGIE for varices* and simultaneously ask for viral serology.
- *If SBC+, refer for transplant.*

Surgery for OCH entails:
- Cholecystectomy, CBD exploration (CBDE), intrahepatic stone clearance (with cholangioscopy or with Fogarty/small foleys bulb)
- If AHC+, multiple intrahepatic strictures, high stone load, with recurrent episodes of cholangitis, plan for resection of that segment (after evaluation of patient comorbidities, PS and liver function)
- Along with Roux-en-Y hepaticojejunostomy (HJ) +/− Access loop if required (depends upon IR expertise for PTBD/accessing jejunal loop percutaneously and comfort/expertise of the endoscopist for gastric access loop)

For follow-up: Do as per follow-up of any HJ—with USG and LFTs and grade as per McDonald's criteria.

■ CHOLEDOCHAL CYST (CDC)

Diagnosis

For CDC evaluation, USG followed by MRCP is enough.

How to diagnose CDC on imaging:
Disproportionate/focal dilatation of bile ducts with sudden proximal tapering, i.e., without peripheral IHBRD, along with distal tapering, seen without any distal obstruction, or even if this picture is seen with distal obstruction, but the dilatation persists even after removal of distal obstruction, then it points to CDC.

Also look for presence of APBDJ (union of MPD and CBD outside the Duodenal wall OR common channel ≥15 mm) and site of insertion of MPD (below or into cyst). Remember that Forme Fruste CDC has APBDJ without much ductal dilatation.

A large Japanese study concluded that preventive cholecystectomy should be done in patients with APBDJ even without ductal dilatation, while rest of the biliary tree must be kept on follow-up.

So now how to differentiate between type 1 and 4A CDC: SGPGI group says that type 1 and 4A CDC, both can involve extra hepatic as well as intrahepatic ducts (RHD and LHD). They say that type 4A CDC will always have a stricture or septum between RHD and LHD which will be seen on preoperative imaging and should be taken care of during surgery, by seeing it with intraoperative cholangioscope and dividing the septum (treatment of choice for both being extra hepatic cyst excision with Roux-en-Y HJ, without excision of RHD and LHD, so life-long follow-up required for intrahepatic part of cyst), otherwise LHD and RHD would not be get decompressed, whereas RHD and LHD dilatation is continuous with extrahepatic ductal dilatation in type 1.

Others strictly label type 1 CDC as involving only extrahepatic ducts, whereas CDC involving extra and intrahepatic (LHD and RHD) ducts as

CHAPTER 3.3: Hepatopancreatobiliary—Management of Cases besides Gallbladder Cancer

type 4A. Also in type 4A if one sided intrahepatic ducts are grossly dilated, then that sided hepatectomy can be added to extra hepatic cyst excision with Roux-en-Y HJ.

So always in MRCP of CDC, look at upper end for above controversy and also to look for any aberrant right sectoral entering cyst which is seen more commonly in CDC (and must be safeguarded or must be drained as a separate anastomosis) as per SGPGI group, and also look for lower end to look for APBDJ and to see where MPD is entering (into cyst or below it) to know lower end of excision.

If malignancy is suspected in CDC (which will look like a papillary intraluminal growth), then do CECT as well.

Surgical Tips for CDC (Box 1)

- *During CDC surgery, it can be adherent to PV, at that time use Lillys technique* where posterior wall is left behind and mucosa can be destroyed.
- *Upper end of CDC transection*: Just few mm below the Hilum, leaving a cuff of CHD behind (for HJ) and ductotomy should be extended to anterior aspect of LHD as well.
- *Lower end of CDC transection*: When cyst starts to taper, above MPD. (Look for MRCP findings, so if the cyst is terminating well above MPD, complete excision is possible, but if MPD is terminating into cyst, part of cyst has to be left behind otherwise MPD will get injured, and then remnant cyst wall of anterior, posterior and lateral sides can be destroyed, but not medial wall, to safeguard MPD. So the cyst left behind, has chance of malignancy and needs life-long follow-up)

Box 1: Todani modification of Alonso Lej classification and its management in brief.[44]

- Type 1: Solitary extrahepatic cyst
  - Excision with Roux-en-Y hepaticojejunostomy (HJ)
- Type 2: Extrahepatic supraduodenal diverticula
  - Excision with Roux-en-Y HJ
- Type 3: Choledochocele: intraduodenal diverticula
  - Surgical transduodenal excision
- Type 4:
  - A: Multiple extrahepatic and intrahepatic cysts
    - For extrahepatic component: Excision with Roux-en-Y HJ
    - For intrahepatic component: Hepatic resection
  - B: Multiple extrahepatic cysts
    - Excision with Roux-en-Y HJ
- Type 5: Caroli disease: Multiple intrahepatic cysts
  - Liver transplant
- Type 6: Isolated dilatation of cystic duct
  - Excision

- *If MPD gets injured,* then it can be reimplanted, or intraoperative ERCP and MPD stenting can be done across and MPD repaired over it, and if ERCP not available, then do a duodenotomy, try to cannulate MPD with a guidewire, cross the injury site and then put a pancreatic stent across and repair the MPD over it. As a last resort pancreaticoduodenectomy (PD) may have to be done.

■ MANAGEMENT OF CHOLEDOCHOLITHIASIS

Options available:
- Preoperative ERCP with biliary stone clearance and stenting followed by laparoscopic cholecystectomy followed by biliary stent removal
- Laparoscopic CBD exploration and cholecystectomy: Transcystic or trans-choledochal
- Open CBD exploration and cholecystectomy

■ REFERENCES

1. Ngamruengphong S, Bartel MJ, Raimondo M. Cyst carcinoembryonic antigen in differentiating pancreatic cysts: a meta-analysis. Dig Liver Dis. 2013;45(11):920-6.
2. Brugge WR, Lewandrowski K, Lee-Lewandrowski E, Centeno BA, Szydlo T, Regan S, et al. Diagnosis of pancreatic cystic neoplasms: a report of the cooperative pancreatic cyst study. Gastroenterology. 2004;126(5):1330-6.
3. Faias S, Cravo M, Chaves P, Pereira L. Comparative analysis of glucose and carcinoembryonic antigen in the diagnosis of pancreatic mucinous cysts: a systematic review and meta-analysis. Gastrointest Endosc. 2021;94(2):235-47.
4. Van der Waaij LA, van Dullemen HM, Porte RJ. Cyst fluid analysis in the differential diagnosis of pancreatic cystic lesions: a pooled analysis. Gastrointest Endosc. 2005;62(3):383-9.
5. McCarty TR, Paleti S, Rustagi T. Molecular analysis of EUS-acquired pancreatic cyst fluid for KRAS and GNAS mutations for diagnosis of intraductal papillary mucinous neoplasia and mucinous cystic lesions: a systematic review and meta-analysis. Gastrointest Endosc. 2021;93(5):1019-1033.e5.
6. Singhi AD, McGrath K, Brand RE, Khalid A, Zeh HJ, Chennat JS, et al. Preoperative next-generation sequencing of pancreatic cyst fluid is highly accurate in cyst classification and detection of advanced neoplasia. Gut. 2018;67(12):2131-41.
7. Springer S, Wang Y, Molin MD, Masica DL, Jiao Y, Kinde I, et al. A combination of molecular markers and clinical features improve the classification of pancreatic cysts. Gastroenterology. 2015;149(6):1501-10.
8. Sureka B, Bihari C, Arora A, Agrawal N, Bharathy KG, Dev K, et al. Imaging paradigm of cystic lesions in pancreas. JOP. J Pancreas (Online). 2016;17(5):452-65.
9. Elta GH, Enestvedt BK, Sauer BG, Lennon AM. ACG clinical guideline: diagnosis and management of pancreatic cysts. Am J Gastroenterol. 2018;113(4):464-79.
10. Verbeke CS, Hauge T. European evidence-based guidelines on pancreatic cystic neoplasms European Study Group on Cystic Tumours of the Pancreas. Gut. 2018;67(5):789-804.
11. Tanaka M, Fernández-del Castillo C, Kamisawa T, Jang JY, Levy P, Ohtsuka T, et al. Revisions of international consensus Fukuoka guidelines for the management of IPMN of the pancreas. Pancreatology. 2017;17(5):738-53.
12. Law JK, Ahmed A, Singh VK, Akshintala VS, Olson MT, Raman SP, et al. A systematic review of solid-pseudopapillary neoplasms: are these rare lesions?. Pancreas. 2014;43(3):331-7.
13. Megibow AJ, Baker ME, Morgan DE, Kamel IR, Sahani DV, Newman E, et al. Management of incidental pancreatic cysts: a white paper of the ACR Incidental Findings Committee. J Am Coll Radiol. 2017;14(7):911-23.

14. Nougaret S, Reinhold C, Chong J, Escal L, Mercier G, Fabre JM, et al. Incidental pancreatic cysts: natural history and diagnostic accuracy of a limited serial pancreatic cyst MRI protocol. Eur Radiol. 2014;24:1020-9.
15. Gil E, Choi SH, Choi DW, Heo JS, Kim MJ. Mucinous cystic neoplasms of the pancreas with ovarian stroma. ANZ J Surg. 2013;83(12):985-90.
16. Bałdys-Waligórska A, Nowak A. Neuroendocrine neoplasms of the digestive system-current classification and terminology. Biuletyn Polskiego Towarzystwa Onkologicznego Nowotwory. 2021;6(1):26-37.
17. Vinik AI, Chaya C. Clinical presentation and diagnosis of neuroendocrine tumors. Hematol Oncol Clin North Am. 2016;30(1):21-48.
18. Modlin IM, Kidd M, Bodei L, Drozdov I, Aslanian H. The clinical utility of a novel blood-based multi-transcriptome assay for the diagnosis of neuroendocrine tumors of the gastrointestinal tract. Am J Gastroenterol. 2015;110(8):1223-32.
19. Reubi JC. Somatostatin and other Peptide receptors as tools for tumor diagnosis and treatment. Neuroendocrinology . 2004:80 Suppl 1:51-6.
20. Treglia G, Castaldi P, Rindi G, Giordano A, Rufini V. Diagnostic performance of Gallium-68 somatostatin receptor PET and PET/CT in patients with thoracic and gastroenteropancreatic neuroendocrine tumours: a meta-analysis. Endocrine. 2012;42:80-7.
21. Puli SR, Kalva N, Bechtold ML, Pamulaparthy SR, Cashman MD, Estes NC, et al. Diagnostic accuracy of endoscopic ultrasound in pancreatic neuroendocrine tumors: a systematic review and meta analysis. World J Gastroenterol. 2013;19(23):3678.
22. Kuo JH, Lee JA, Chabot JA. Nonfunctional pancreatic neuroendocrine tumors. Surg Clin North Am. 2014;94(3):689-708.
23. Morgan RE, Pommier SJ, Pommier RF. Expanded criteria for debulking of liver metastasis also apply to pancreatic neuroendocrine tumors. Surgery. 2018;163(1):218-25.
24. Finkelstein P, Sharma R, Picado O, Gadde R, Stuart H, Ripat C, et al. Pancreatic neuroendocrine tumors (panNETs): analysis of overall survival of nonsurgical management versus surgical resection. J Gastrointest Surg. 2017;21(5):855-66.
25. Kulke MH, Anthony LB, Bushnell DL, De Herder WW, Goldsmith SJ, Klimstra DS, et al. NANETS treatment guidelines: well-differentiated neuroendocrine tumors of the stomach and pancreas. Pancreas. 2010;39(6):735-52.
26. Falconi M, Bartsch DK, Eriksson B, Klöppel G, Lopes JE, O'connor JM, et al. ENETS Consensus Guidelines for the management of patients with digestive neuroendocrine neoplasms of the digestive system: well-differentiated pancreatic non-functioning tumors. Neuroendocrinology. 2012;95(2):120-34.
27. Jilesen AP, van Eijck CH, Busch OR, van Gulik TM, Gouma DJ, van Dijkum EJ. Postoperative outcomes of enucleation and standard resections in patients with a pancreatic neuroendocrine tumor. World J Surg. 2016;40:715-28.
28. Falconi M, Eriksson B, Kaltsas G, Bartsch DK, Capdevila J, Caplin M, et al. ENETS consensus guidelines update for the management of patients with functional pancreatic neuroendocrine tumors and non-functional pancreatic neuroendocrine tumors. Neuroendocrinology. 2016;103(2):153-71.
29. Kunz PL, Reidy-Lagunes D, Anthony LB, Bertino EM, Brendtro K, Chan JA, et al. Consensus guidelines for the management and treatment of neuroendocrine tumors. Pancreas. 2013;42(4):557-77.
30. Riihimäki M, Hemminki A, Sundquist K, Sundquist J, Hemminki K. The epidemiology of metastases in neuroendocrine tumors. Int J Cancer. 2016;139(12):2679-86.
31. Moris D, Tsilimigras DI, Ntanasis-Stathopoulos I, Beal EW, Felekouras E, Vernadakis S, et al. Liver transplantation in patients with liver metastases from neuroendocrine tumors: A systematic review. Surgery. 2017;162(3):525-36.
32. Almond LM, Hodson J, Ford SJ, Gourevitch D, Roberts KJ, Shah T, et al. Role of palliative resection of the primary tumour in advanced pancreatic and small intestinal neuro-endocrine tumours: a systematic review and meta-analysis. Eur J Surg Oncol. 2017;43(10):1808-15.

33. Yoshida T, Hijioka S, Hosoda W, Ueno M, Furukawa M, Kobayashi N, et al. Surgery for pancreatic neuroendocrine tumor G3 and carcinoma G3 should be considered separately. Ann Surg Oncol. 2019;26:1385-93.
34. Gragerov AI, Danilevskaya ON, Didichenko SA, Kaverina EN. An ARS element from Drosophila melanogaster telomeres contains the yeast ARS core and bent replication enhancer. Nucleic Acids Research. 1988;16(3):1169-80.
35. Pieterman CR, De Laat JM, Twisk JW, Van Leeuwaarde RS, de Herder WW, Dreijerink KM, et al. Long-term natural course of small nonfunctional pancreatic neuroendocrine tumors in MEN1—results from the Dutch MEN1 Study Group. J Clin Endocrinol Metab. 2017;102(10):3795-805.
36. Partelli S, Tamburrino D, Lopez C, Albers M, Milanetto AC, Pasquali C, et al. Active surveillance versus surgery of nonfunctioning pancreatic neuroendocrine neoplasms ≤ 2 cm in MEN1 patients. Neuroendocrinology. 2016;103(6):779-86.
37. Kennedy AS. Hepatic-directed Therapies in Patients with Neuroendocrine Tumors. Hematol Oncol Clin North Am. 2016;30(1):193-207.
38. Leung DA, Goin JE, Sickles C, Raskay BJ, Soulen MC. Determinants of postembolization syndrome after hepatic chemoembolization. J Vasc Interv Radiol . 2001;12(3):321-6.
39. Raymond E, Dahan L, Raoul JL, Bang YJ, Borbath I, Lombard-Bohas C, er al. Sunitinib malate for the treatment of pancreatic neuroendocrine tumors. N Engl J Med. 2011;364(6):501-13.
40. Yao JC, Shah MH, Ito T, Bohas CL, Wolin EM, Van Cutsem E, et al. Everolimus for advanced pancreatic neuroendocrine tumors. N Engl J Med. 2011;364(6):514-23.
41. Ramirez RA, Beyer DT, Chauhan A, Boudreaux JP, Wang YZ, Woltering EA. The role of capecitabine/temozolomide in metastatic neuroendocrine tumors. The Oncologist. 2016;21(6):671-5.
42. Strosberg J, El-Haddad G, Wolin E, Hendifar A, Yao J, Chasen B, et al. Phase 3 trial of 177Lu-Dotatate for midgut neuroendocrine tumors. N Eng J Med. 2017;376(2):125-35.
43. Garcia-Carbonero R, Rinke A, Valle JW, Fazio N, Caplin M, Gorbounova V, et al. ENETS Consensus Guidelines for the Standards of Care in Neuroendocrine Neoplasms. Systemic Therapy 2: Chemotherapy. Neuroendocrinology. 2017;105(3):281-94.
44. Todani T, Watanabe Y, Narusue M, Tabuchi K, Okajima K. Congenital bile duct cysts: classification, operative procedures, and review of thirty-seven cases including cancer arising from choledochal cyst. Am J Surg. 1977;134(2):263-9.

3.4 CHAPTER

Hepatopancreatobiliary— Gallbladder Cancer Management

SGPGI Lucknow, GB Pant Delhi, PGI Chandigarh, AIIMS Delhi, and TMH Mumbai, have contributed immensely to this field. The following discussion is based on the teachings from these institutions.

■ DIAGNOSIS, EVALUATION AND TERMINOLOGIES

CXR, USG abdomen to be done for all cases. If CXR shows cannonball metastases, then no further investigations are needed and it makes the intent of treatment palliative.

If on USG, suspicious lesion in gallbladder (GB) (intraluminal polypoidal lesion/ focal irregular non-uniform wall thickening/mass replacing GB or focal stippled mucosal calcification of porcelain GB), follow it up with all blood tests, *CA 19-9 (cancer antigen 19-9), and then CECT chest/abdomen/pelvis to be done.*

If it is a papillary tumor in GB, or if it is a gallbladder cancer (GBC) neck with jaundice, or if there's sludge/calculi seen in GB, deranged LFT, and there's dilated common bile duct (CBD), always ask for MRI with MRCP as it may significantly change management. GBC with any amount of liver infiltration at neck and infiltrating hilum: Extended right hepatectomy (ERH)/modified ERH with CBD excision. GBC with CBD infiltration and also tumor emboli from a papillary tumor: CBD excision. Disproportionate bile duct dilatation without peripheral *IHBRD* in situation of no/insignificant distal obstruction like a small calculus OR persistence of dilatation even post-ERCP stenting, points to it being a choledochal cyst (CDC) and requires CBD excision as well. Whereas calculi in CBD require preoperative therapeutic ERCP with clearance/stenting.

Also, if the tumor is locally advanced, or if ERH/HPD is planned, then FDG PET CT is a must to rule out distant disease.

NACT can be considered as per Tata Memorial Hospital, Mumbai (TMH) protocol (which requires tissue diagnosis and complete staging with PET CT and staging laparoscopy before starting chemotherapy).

After NACT, repeat FDG PET CT (for restaging and to assess response) *and staging laparoscopy* (just before laparotomy for definitive surgery, to rule out metastases).

So before surgery, staging laparoscopy is to be done for all GBC patients (if any deposit, then send for frozen, and if positive, then abandon) followed by exploratory laparotomy with a thorough intraoperative assessment for deposits, followed by Kocherization and interaortocaval (IAC) node sampling OR Celiac/SMA node sampling (this part can be done laparoscopically also, depends on expertise) and frozen (if positive, abandon), followed by cystic duct margin for frozen (if positive, add CBD excision to extended cholecystectomy, and then CBD upper and lower margins also need to be sent for frozen, and procedure is modified accordingly as given below).

Types based on timing of GBC detection as defined by Professor VK Kapoor (VKK) in his seminal work on GBC from India:
- *Obvious*: RHC dull continuous pain, jaundice, hard mass palpated with ascites, etc.
- *Suspected*: Preoperative imaging showing thick walled GB (TWGB) defined by wall thickness (WT) ≥4 mm, polyp or mass
- *Unsuspected*: Intraoperative findings of TWGB/difficult dissection or on opening GB—nodule, polyp, ulcer seen. GB is sent for frozen always in this scenario
- *Missed*: Either GB was not sent for histopathological exam (HPE) because it looked grossly normal, OR it was missed by pathologist on HPE as well
- *Incidental*: Diagnosed for the first time on HPE.

■ MANAGEMENT IN BRIEF

Indian "Middle Path" or the "Buddhist Approach" to GBC given by Professor VKK, balancing the Japanese aggressive approach with the western nihilism toward GBC. So aggressive approach to early GBC and conservative approach to advanced GBC is the essence of the Buddhist Approach. The management principles for various GBC scenarios as per this approach are as follows:
- *For preoperative diagnosis of T1aN0 disease, (only if confirmed by EUS)*: Full thickness cholecystectomy is a procedure (Rarely done).
  However, in a more common situation, T1a is a diagnosis post-cholecystectomy done for gallstone disease (GSD), and must be approached as per "incidental GBC" section below.
- *For preoperative diagnosis of TWGB with low suspicion of GBC (Preoperative imaging showing uniformly TWGB)—Only 3% turn out to be cancer (CA)*
  OR
- *For intraoperative unsuspected finding of TWGB/difficult calots dissection*: Anticipatory extended cholecystectomy (AEC with 1 cm liver wedge, as defined by Professor VKK aka the Lucknow approach) to be done and sent for frozen. If positive, then do the lymphadenectomy.
  And also if mass/polyp/thickening found on opening specimen, send it for frozen. If malignancy positive, then completion extended cholecystectomy (CEC) to be done.

- *Whereas for preoperative diagnosis of a TWGB with high suspicion of GBC* (Intraluminal mass or focal irregular non-uniform thickening or mass replacing GB), upfront *extended cholecystectomy (EC) is the procedure of choice (Discussed in detail after "incidental GBC" section).*
- *For incidental GBC:*
  - If a simple cholecystectomy was done for presumed GSD, and postoperative biopsy comes to be T1a (without involvement of the Rokitansky-Aschoff sinuses) and cystic duct margin and cystic node is negative (remember cystic LN is not sentinel in GBC), lymphovascular invasion (LVI), perineural invasion (PNI) negative *and* finally if specimen was intact and there was no bile spill, *only then* simple cholecystectomy is curative. However, if any of these criteria are not fulfilled, then CEC must be done.
  - In every case, try to find out from primary surgeon if there was perforation/bile spill, if bag used to remove specimen, which port used to remove specimen. And review HPE (T, N, cystic duct margin, LVI, PNI).

    This is because perforation/bile spill are poor prognostic factors, and increase chance of port site dissemination (All ports have equal risk. Also, port sites may get involved even without these in GBC, due to pneumoperitoneum, gas currents). If bag is used, it may at most reduce risk of metastases to that port, but other ports are still at risk.

    Also, LVI, PNI, are poor prognostic factors, so for all of these above, NACT must be given.
  - *Before CEC, do complete staging as is done before EC*, including FDG PET CT (to be done after 4–6 weeks of index surgery) and staging lap.
  - *CEC: Best results if done between 4–8 weeks of index procedure*, so disease gets time to show it is biology, as poor biology disease will show *metastasis* and it would have been futile to operate early in them.
  - *NACT should be given in this waiting period in case of presence of high-risk features for recurrence, as given by TMH protocol* (Residual/recurrent disease in GB fossa, Type 1/2 biliary block, regional LN present) to select good biology disease.
  - *NACT must also be given if there was perforation/bile spill during the index surgery or if specimen shows LVI, PNI, as discussed*
  - So during surgery for CEC, staging laparoscopy and same protocol to be followed as for EC (given on top). If bag was not used for extraction, and if only the extraction port site (epigastric/umbilical) is positive for disease without any other peritoneal/metastatic disease spread (as seen on preoperative CECT/FDG PET CT), then it is only local disease and port excision will add to survival. However, if port is positive along with presence of peritoneal disease, then it is metastatic disease and excision would not be add to OS, however it may only help in reducing local pain of infiltration if it is there and to stage the disease. Many groups including MSKCC do not advise routine port site excision, whereas SGPGI group routinely advocates full thickness skin to peritoneum excision of all port sites.

- *Adjuvant chemotherapy must be given in all GBC having ≥T2, N+, positive margin, papillary tumor, poorly differentiated and LVI, PNI, along with those who had bile spill during the index cholecystectomy.* Despite its limitations, the *BILCAP* trial has defined the standard of care adjuvant therapy after re-resection of incidental GBC to be 6 months of capecitabine. This recommendation is regardless of margin or lymph node status, and has been endorsed by ASCO.

  Also, in R1 positive GBC, SWOG 0809 regimen recommended by NCCN and ASCO as adjuvant CRT: *4#GEMCAP followed by RT* (45 Gy to LN region and 50–54 Gy to tumor bed).

  However, if NACT of a particular kind was given already (e.g., *GEMCIS or GEMOX as per TMH* protocol), then the same chemotherapy must be given as adjuvant, for a total of 6 months of perioperative chemotherapy.

- *Now discussing preoperative TWGB with high suspicion of GBC in detail*:
  - *So for preoperative TWGB with high suspicion of GBC*: Just remember that if major liver resection is planned, then first FDG PET CT and staging lap must be done to rule out *metastasis*, followed by preoperative biliary drainage *(PBD) of FLR* (if jaundiced due to biliary block), and bilirubin must be brought <3 (although complete hepatic function recovery takes 6 weeks, clinically 2–3 weeks is enough), and if ERH is planned, then PBD must be followed by PVE (once bilirubin comes below 3) of right portal vein (RPV) and segment 4 portal supply for augmentation of FLR, and then if FLR is adequate after 2–3 weeks on repeat imaging, then staging laparoscopy must be repeated to again rule out *metastases*, and only then definitive surgery to be done.
  - NACT may be given in this waiting period after PBD when the bilirubin comes below 3 (after diagnosis is confirmed by EUS FNA), if indicated, as per TMH protocol (T3/4 or Type 1/2 biliary block or Regional LN positive on preoperative imaging).
  - GEMCIS or GEMOX average of 4 cycles, followed by surgery and adjuvant chemotherapy (total of 6 months of perioperative chemotherapy).
  - *If GBC neck is extending into cystic duct/CBD without liver infiltration*: Extended cholecystectomy with CBD excision done from hilum to duodenal end. [Upper and lower ends of CBD sent for frozen in all cases needing CBD excision: So if upper end is positive for malignancy, then it needs right hepatectomy, and if lower end is positive for malignancy, then it needs pancreaticoduodenectomy (PD)]
  - *If GBC neck is extending into cystic duct/CBD*:
    - With liver infiltration ≤1 cm: Classical right hepatectomy with 2 cm wedge resection of segment 4B, along with CBD excision.
    - With liver infiltration >1 cm: Two options—ERH or modified ERH (Classical right hepatectomy plus 4B resection, sparing 4A) along with CBD excision.
      (Remember that the right portal pedicle lies at a depth of only 2–9 mm in the region of GB neck. So any amount of liver infiltration of GBC neck mandates a right hepatectomy, and as 4B forms GB bed, for GBC

it is always ERH/Modified ERH. So now, for liver infiltration ≤1 cm, RH with 4B wedge resection is feasible, but if it is >1 cm, then 4B has to come out, so the only options that remain are ERH and modified ERH) Before ERH, FDG PET CT and staging laparoscopy, followed by PBD of FLR (segments 2 and 3) with right and also segment 4 PVE (only after bilirubin comes to <3) must be done. After 2–3 weeks of PVE, CT volumetry must be done and if FLR is adequate, repeat staging laparoscopy must be done to assess for *metastases* before definitive procedure can be done.

For modified ERH if FLR volume is enough, then no need of PVE, however PBD must always be done whenever any major hepatic resection is planned (≥3 segment resection).

- *For GBC neck extending into hilum (biliary confluence), without liver infiltration*, then central hepatectomy (segments 4, 5, 8 resection) or Taj Mahal resection (1, 4B, 5) can be done, but technically very difficult, and if that's the case, then ERH or modified ERH or RH with at least a wedge resection of 4B will have to be done along with CBD excision.
- *However, if along with hilum, GBC neck is also invading liver (that means right portal pedicle is involved)*, then the only options are ERH/modified ERH or RH with at least a wedge resection of 4B as per similar principles as above.
- *GBC in fundus/body with up to 1 cm liver infiltration*: Extended cholecystectomy
- *GBC in fundus/body with more than 1 cm liver infiltration*: 4B and 5 resection or modified ERH or even ERH may have to be done (*Miyazaki technique* for 4B/5 resection: Ligate inflow to 4B, followed by Right posterior sectoral pedicle ligation for demarcation of 6 from 5, and then horizontal line extended from demarcation of 4 up to 5).
- Central hepatectomy (4, 5, 8 resection) and Taj Mahal resection (1, 4B, 5) can be done for GBC involving hilum, *but not* right portal pedicle, for which, extended right hepatectomy is done.
- Combined resection of adjacent organs, which involves resection of CBD, sleeve resection of duodenum, colon, wedge resection of pancreas (few reports but technical difficulties), HPD (resection of at least ≥3 liver segments with PD), hepato-ligamento-pancreato-duodenectomy (HLPD) and right upper quadrantectomy (including right nephrectomy)
    - *NCCN guidelines recommend* adjuvant 5-FU/gemcitabine-based chemo/chemoRT (chemotherapy plus radiation therapy) for all except T1N0 tumors.
    - *ESMO recommends* adjuvant chemoRT in high-risk cases.
    - *ASCO recommends* adjuvant chemotherapy with capecitabine for 6 months in patients who have undergone resection.
    - *SWOG 0809 recommended* CRT after R1 resection.
- *Non-curative cholecystectomy*: Can be done only if on laparotomy, disease is found to be incurable (distant *metastases*) and preoperative clinical stage is at the most T2. Benefits: Reduces tumor burden, so better effect of

palliative chemoradiotherapy and increase in OS seen. Also morbidity in terms of future attacks of cholecystitis/empyema GB is eliminated.
- *Indication for CBD excision in GBC*:
  - For papillary variant of GBC with tumor emboli spread to within CBD
  - GBC of neck/cystic duct infiltrating into CBD or positive frozen for cystic duct margin
  - For LN densely adherent to CBD
  - For GBC with choledochal cyst
  - Routine CBD excision in anticipation of occult perineural/periductal spread.(Not routinely advocated by most groups, same was proved by the French multicentre trial)
- *Adjuvant chemotherapy trials for biliary CA (GBC/Cholangiocarcinoma)*:
  - *BCAT*: Gemcitabine versus observation
  - *PRODIGE 12/ACCORD 18*: GEMOX versus observation
  - *BILCAP*: Capecitabine
  - *ASCOT (ongoing)*: S1 versus observation

Of these given above, GEM based chemotherapy did not improve OS, but capecitabine improved some outcomes. S1 has shown promise.
- *Adjuvant CRT for R1 positive resected GBC*: SWOG 0809 regimen recommended by NCCN and ASCO in high-risk GBC (pT2-4, LN positive, and positive margins): 4#GEMCAP followed by RT (45 Gy to LN region and 50–54 Gy to tumor bed).
- *Palliative chemotherapy*:
  - *ABC-02 trial*: 6 cycles GEMCIS is better than gemcitabine alone, and improves OS.
  - *ABC-12 study*: GEMCIS plus Durvalumab was approved by NICE in January 2024 as the first line standard of care for those with inoperable GBC or cholangioca.
  - *PRODIGE 38-AMEBICA*: GEMCIS versus mFOLFIRINOX (more toxic). No difference in PFS and OS.

3.5
CHAPTER

Hepatopancreatobiliary— Imaging Lesions

■ LIVER

Liver Protocol Contrast-enhanced Computed Tomography (CECT)
- *Non-contrast*
- *Early arterial*: 18 seconds
- *Late arterial*: 35 seconds
- *Portal venous (PV)*: 65–70 seconds
- *Delayed*: 3–10 minutes

SOLID LIVER LESIONS—BENIGN

Hemangioma:
Hypodense in non-contrast computed tomography (CT).
Enhances progressively in all contrast phases from periphery to center (enhancement pattern same as of vessel in that particular phase, so in arterial phase same like artery and in portal phase same as portal vein) with peripheral globular puddling of contrast in arterial phase, followed by progressive centripetal enhancement in PV and delayed phases.

Focal Nodular Hyperplasia:
Hypodense in non-contrast with central hypodense scar.
Arterial phase homogeneous hyperenhancement (entire lesion lights up in arterial phase except central hypodense scar) and in PV phase lesion becomes isoenhancing but never hypoenhancing, with delayed enhancement of central scar.

Adenoma:
Hypodense in non-contrast due to fat/old bleed/necrosis OR may be hyperdense due to fresh bleed/excess glycogen.

Arterial phase hyperenhancing [but lesser than focal nodular hyperplasia (FNH)] and no scar, rest same like FNH.

(*Three main types*: Hepatocyte nuclear factor (HNF) 1 alpha seen in type 1 with MODY and glycogen storage disorders, beta catenin type 2 associated with males, steroids, malignancy, inflammatory type 3 associated with raised IL-6, TNF-alpha, CRP. Adenomas are prone to rupture, bleed, cause pain, fever and cancer).

SOLID LIVER LESIONS—MALIGNANT
Fibrolamellar Hepatocellular Carcinoma
Hypodense in non-contrast with coarse calcifications in central scar. Remember background liver will be normal.
Lesion is arterial phase heterogeneously hyperenhancing, with atypical washout in PV phase, majority isoenhancing, with few being hyper/hypoenhancing.

In most the central scar does not enhance, but in a few it may have persistent enhancement in delayed phase.

HCC
Hypodense in non-contrast due to necrosis/fat or heterogeneous.

LIRADS 5 in a cirrhotic liver:
In a cirrhotic liver, for a lesion ≥ 2 cm having *non-rim* arterial phase hyperenhancement, presence of ≥ 1 of the following major criteria is diagnostic of HCC:
1. Non-peripheral PV washout, becoming hypoenhancing
2. Enhancing capsule in PV/delayed phase (seen in >90% which are ≥ 5 cm, in Asians)
3. Threshold growth (>5 mm and >50% increase <6 months or >100% increase in >6 months, OR new lesion >10 mm in <24 months)

And for a lesion 10–19 mm, along with APHE, ≥ 2 other major criteria must be present to be diagnosed as HCC in a cirrhotic liver.

Intrahepatic Cholangiocarcinoma (IHCC)
Hypodense/heterogeneous in non-contrast with subcapsular retraction seen. Peripheral rim enhancement with an overall hypoenhancing lesion in arterial phase which enhances progressively (non-globular) in PV phase with central pooling of contrast in delayed phase.

NET
Hyperenhancing in arterial phase, with enhancement persistent in venous phase. Mosaic, ring, target enhancement of liver lesion in arterial phase with peripheral washout in PV phase is mostly due to hypervascular secondaries (NET more likely, secondaries from RCC, sarcoma) OR atypical HCC/intrahepatic HCC (IHCC).
While, metastases from other GI cancers show weak peripheral rim enhancement in arterial phase and are hypoenhancing in PV phase.

Cystic Liver Lesions can be Infective or Non-infective

- *Infective*: Amebic liver abscess (ALA), pyogenic liver abscess (PLA), fungal abscess and hydatid cyst.
- *Non Infective*:
    - Benign: Simple cyst, polycystic liver disease (PCLD), biliary hamartoma (Von Meyenburg complex)
    - Premalignant: Choledochal cyst (CDC), Caroli's, mucinous cystic neoplasm-Liver (MCN-L), intraductal papillary mucinous neoplasm (IPMN-B)
    - Malignant: Cystic metastases (from colorectal cancer-CRC/ovarian), cystic HCC, cystic NET, biliary cystadenocarcinoma (BCAC)
    - Traumatic: Biloma, seroma, hematoma

Cystic lesion in liver with internal septae, DDs:
- ALA (enhancing septae, double target sign formed by peripheral enhancing rim and perilesional edema)
- PLA (enhancing septae, conglomerated lesion)
- Hydatid cyst (*septae don't enhance*, no mural nodules. May rupture into duct, which will be seen on MRI)
- MCN-L (thickened wall with papillary growth, mural nodules +, enhancing septae, mostly no communication with duct)
- IPMN-B (multicystic appearance, enhancing cyst walls, may be multifocal, communication with duct +, intraductal masses/nodules in duct, grossly dilated duct due to mucin)
- Cystic metastases/cystic HCC/cystic NET
- BCAC (features of MCN/IPMN, *along with* solid components)

Internal septae represent undigested biliary radicles and Glissonean sheath and enhance in all, whereas in hydatid cyst they are infective septae and hence, do not enhance.

■ LIVER SPACE OCCUPYING LESION (SOL)—TO BIOPSY OR NOT

Liver Primary

If USG, contrast-enhanced computed tomography (CECT) or/and MRI (discuss 1st imaging with radiologist before going for 2nd). Also, both imaging are compulsory for HCC in non-cirrhotic liver as LIRADS do not apply. Also both need to be done for any lesion, when first imaging is inconclusive for it) and available blood tests, serologies, tumor markers are 100% typical/diagnostic of the lesion, *then no need of biopsy, just go ahead with FDG PET/DOTATATE if indicated followed by staging laparoscopy.*

But even after doing all possible blood tests and CECT and MRI both, diagnosis is inconclusive.

- Then for a solid lesion, get biopsy done (EUS guided preferred over transcutaneous), followed by IHC for definitive diagnosis followed by DOTATATE PET if it is NET, or FDG PET only if indicated (like if tumor markers are very

high or extended resection/transplant has to be done), followed by staging laparoscopy/laparotomy and biopsy if all previous efforts futile.
- *But for a cystic lesion, you should not do biopsy.* Because if it is hydatid, it will spill and cause anaphylaxis/dissemination, and If it is a premalignant/malignant cystic tumor, then it will lead to spillage and dissemination.

Then in such a case, if history is not suggestive of an infection like ALA/PLA/hydatid cyst, then either can directly go for anatomical resection and then see postoperative biopsy, OR if patient can afford, go for dual scan (FDG PET and DOTATATE PET), so that at least there is a chance to rule out ADENOCA OR NET, and then proceed accordingly.

For Liver Secondaries

Biopsy is generally needed to proceed with treatment, along with FDG PET/DOTATATE PET as per clinical suspicion.

PANCREAS

Pancreatic Protocol CT

Water as a neutral oral contrast is used to distend the stomach and the duodenum. 100–120 mL of iodinated contrast is injected at a rate of 3–5 mL/s.
- Pancreatic protocol CT-phasing (in seconds):
  - Non-contrast, 17–25 early arterial, 25–35 late arterial (aka pancreatic parenchymal phase), 55–70 portal venous (PV).
  - Slice thickness is 1 mm.
  - Pancreatic cancers are hypoenhancing in pancreatic parenchymal phase. In this phase we also assess the relation of the tumor to the arterial vessels.
  - Similarly, the relation of the tumor to the SMV-PV is evaluated in the PV phase (also useful to see liver metastases) and tumor becomes isoenhancing in the PV phase.

Pancreatic AdenoCA

- Hypo- to iso-dense in noncontrast.
- Hypoenhancing in late arterial (aka pancreatic parenchymal phase).
- Isoenhancing in the PV phase.
  (A large pancreatic mass apart from adenoCA can be lymphoma or TB. So always take EUS guided biopsy if possible, before any treatment).

Pancreatic NET

Hyperenhancing in arterial and PV phases.

Pancreatic Cystic Neoplasms

Enhancing septae, solid components, nodules seen after IV contrast administration.

WHAT ALL TO SEE IN DIFFERENT PHASES OF CT

- *Noncontrast*: Comment about lung/pleural nodules, pleural effusion, lung bases. Then about liver surface if it is smooth or irregular/nodular, gross size, any hypodense lesion with septae, any calcification/hemorrhage seen within, any cysts seen. Also compare it's attenuation with spleen (lower attenuation in fatty liver). Look for same things in other organs like GB, pancreas, spleen, kidneys. Look for any radio-opaque calculi in GB, any stent in CBD/MPD, any Ryles tube in stomach.
  In stomach, see if any contrast (neutral/positive) given, distended or not, and then if any distended bowel loops seen.
  Then lastly look for any pelvic cysts and free fluid.
- *Early arterial*: Look from top of liver to the aorta and then from aorta, trace celiac and its branches and then SMA and it's branches. Look for aberrant vessels, any thrombosis, any segment which is not getting filled/passing through a suspected lesion, any pseudoaneurysms.
- *Late arterial*: Look from top of liver, for any enhancing SOLs, then look for any lesions in GB, pancreas (hypoenhancing-adenoCA, hyperenhancing-NET), spleen, and hollow organs. Look at relationship of tumor with vessels. Also comment on how rest of the liver, pancreas is appearing.
- *Portal venous*: Look from top of liver for SOL characterization [progressively enhancing-hemangioma (globular), cholangio CA (non-globular) or hypoenhancing-metastases or washout-HCC], then exact segments involved, then lesion characterization in other organs and relationship with SMV, SV, PV, HV. Any venous thrombosis/filling defects. Look for any collaterals, splenomegaly.
  Also comment on how rest of the liver, pancreas is appearing.

SO HOW TO READ CT AND PROCEED FOR COMPLETE DIAGNOSIS AND STAGING

Please mention everything while reading imaging, whether it is present or not, because even the negative findings are as important.

After finishing the non-contrast phase and mentioning about any lung/pleural nodules and effusion, liver surface and contour, caudate lobe size, fissural widening, any hypodense lesions, calcification, hemorrhage, ascites and early arterial phase for arterial anatomy and pseudoaneurysms, move on to the delayed arterial and PV phases:

So, for any liver/GB/pancreatic lesion:
- *First describe the lesion*: Always describe the approx site, size, shape, surface, wall thickness, enhancement pattern, any internal septa and their enhancement pattern, any solid components inside, or any mural nodules seen, and if it is causing ductal dilatation, any IHBRD (central or even peripheral, with peripheral IHBRD signifying a significant downstream obstruction) and atrophy hypertrophy complex (AHC)

- Then relationship of the lesion with major vessels (artery and PV/SMV/SV/IVC), any venous thrombosis, collaterals—presence of Cavernoma, also portal cavernoma cholangiopathy (PCC) leading to dilated ducts, splenomegaly, and also relationship with surrounding organs/diaphragmatic crura, etc.
- Followed by regional nodes, distant nodes, omental, peritoneal, pelvic deposits and ascites.
- Then ask for any further investigations if needed, for better characterization of lesion and also to see ductal system like MRI with MRCP, (always mention about IHBRD whether present or not- so right or left sided signifies obstruction on that side respectively, whereas, central/bilateral signifies obstruction at the confluence/CHD/CBD, then always mention about AHC whether present or not: Crowding of ducts irrespective of dilatation signifies atrophy on that side, with elongated and widely spread out ducts on contralateral side signifying compensatory hypertrophy, any intraductal lesions), along with diffusion weighted MRI (DW-MRI) for suspected liver metastases, EUS (for better characterization of lesion with its detailed description, location, and relationship with vessels) and EUS FNA (fluid analysis, cytology, biopsy and IHC), ERCP/PTC with cholangioscopy and biopsy, etc.
- Finally for M staging/assessing metabolic response, FDG PET CT or DOTATATE CT if needed. Try to get a confirmed diagnosis 100% before any treatment.
- Then plan if after staging laparoscopy, you will go for NACT/downstaging by other methods OR upfront surgery.

■ MR IMAGING—BASIC UNDERSTANDING OF SOME TERMINOLOGIES

- Fat is bright on T1 and T2
- Water (CSF, BILE) is bright only on T2
- All IV contrast MR images by default are T1 fat suppressed, *whereas MRCP*, which uses bile itself as contrast is a heavily T2 weighted image.
  In heavily T2 weighted images, metastases lose signal, while signal persists in hemangiomas.
- Fat suppression means that the (white) signal from fat is suppressed, so that lesions that enhance after giving IV contrast can be visualized without fat signals interfering
- Fat saturation is one method for fat suppression, so essentially fat saturated and fat suppressed/attenuated mean the same
- *Meaning of in phase and out of phase (IP-OOP)*: Because water and fat protons have slightly different resonance frequencies, their spins go in- and out-of-phase with each other as a function of time. This phase cancellation effect could be used clinically to identify and even quantify the fat content of tissues like the liver. One particularly common use of this principle today is to help in the differentiation of adrenal adenomas (that typically contain fat) from carcinomas and metastases (that do not). The diagnosis of a variety of other abdominal lesions, including angiomyolipomas, renal clear cell carcinoma, and focal fatty infiltration of the liver may be assisted by IP-OOP imaging.

3.6 CHAPTER

Hepatopancreatobiliary—Ward

Candidate must be familiar with the known postoperative major complications of Hepatopancreatobiliary (HPB) surgery, like posthepatectomy hemorrhage (PHH), posthepatectomy liver failure (PHLF), *biliary leak*, postoperative pancreatic fistula (POPF), postpancreatectomy hemorrhage (PPH), postpancreatectomy acute pancreatitis (PPAP) along with their standard definitions and management protocols.

■ POSTHEPATECTOMY COMPLICATIONS

Posthepatectomy Hemorrhage (Table 1)[1]

Causes

Early:
- Hepatic venous outflow tract obstruction (HVOTO) due to kink and increase in back pressure, slipped ligature, raw surface.
- Coagulopathy due to: prolonged ischemia, >4L transfusions and sepsis from infected bile spill.

TABLE 1: ISGLS definition and severity grading of posthepatectomy hemorrhage (PHH)	
Definition	PHH is defined as a drop of hemoglobin level >3 g/dL after the end of surgery compared to postoperative baseline level and/or any postoperative transfusion of PRBCs for a falling hemoglobin and/or the need for invasive re-intervention (e.g., embolization or re-laparotomy) to stop bleeding
	To diagnose PHH (and to exclude other sources of hemorrhage) evidence of intra-abdominal bleeding should be obtained such as frank blood loss via the abdominal drains if present (e.g., hemoglobin level in drain fluid >3 g/dL) or detection of an intra-abdominal hematoma or active hemorrhage by abdominal imaging (ultrasound, CT, angiography). Patients who are transfused immediately postoperatively for intra-operative blood loss by a maximum of two units of PRBCs (i.e., who do not have evidence of active hemorrhage) are not diagnosed with PHH
Grading	A PHH requiring transfusion of up to 2 units of PRBCs
	B PHH requiring transfusion of >2 units of PRBCs but manageable without invasive intervention
	C PHH requiring radiological interventional treatment (e.g. embolization) or re-laparotomy

Late: Pseudoaneurysms secondary to infected collections.

Indications for intervention:
1. Hemodynamic instability despite adequate resuscitation
2. ≥3 g/dL drop with >3 PRCs given
3. Blood loss >1 L in 8 hours

During surgery: Evacuate clot (persistent presence of clot leads to fibrinolysis), look for source (liver and others). If no source, drain and close.

Posthepatectomy Liver Failure

ISGLS Definition and Grading of Posthepatectomy Liver Failure

In 2011, the International Study Group of Liver Surgery (ISGLS) proposed a standardized definition and severity of grading of PHLF. The consensus conference committee defined PHLF as "a post-operatively acquired deterioration in the ability of the liver to maintain its synthetic, excretory, and detoxifying functions, which are characterized by an increased INR and concomitant hyperbilirubinemia on or after postoperative day 5" **(Table 2)**.[2]

Predictive Factors Associated with Increased Risk of PHLF

Patient Associated

- Age >65 years
- Sex [risk double in males, especially those with hepatocellular carcinoma (HCC)]
- Diabetes mellitus
- Obesity
- Hepatitis B, C
- Malnutrition
- Sepsis
- Renal insufficiency
- Thrombocytopenia
- Lung disease

Liver Associated

- Steatosis (nonalcoholic steatohepatitis and chemotherapy-associated steatohepatitis)
- Fibrosis
- Cirrhosis
- Cholestasis
- Chemotherapy-associated steatohepatitis

Surgery Associated

- Estimated blood loss (EBL) >1,200 mL
- Intraoperative transfusions
- Need for vascular resection

TABLE 2: ISGLS definition and grading of PHLF

Grade	Clinical description	Treatment	Diagnosis	Clinical symptoms	Location for care
A	Deterioration in liver function	None	• UOP >0.5 mL/kg/h • BUN <150 mg/dL • >90% O_2 saturation • INR <1.5	None	Surgical ward
B	Deviation from expected post-operative course without requirement for invasive procedures	Non-invasive: Fresh frozen plasma; albumin; diuretics; non-invasive ventilatory support; abdominal ultrasound; CT scan	• UOP ≤0.5 mL/kg/h • BUN <150 mg/dL • <90% O_2 saturation despite oxygen supplementation • INR ≥1.5, <2.0	• Ascites • Weight gain • Mild respiratory Insufficiency • Confusion • Encephalopathy	Intermediate unit or ICU
C	Multisystem failure requiring invasive treatment	Invasive: Hemodialysis; intubation; extracorporeal liver support; salvage hepatectomy; vasopressors; intravenous glucose for hypoglycemia; ICP monitor	• UOP ≤0.5 mL/kg/h • BUN ≥150 mg/dL • ≤85% O_2 saturation despite high fraction of inspired oxygen support • INR ≥2.0	• Renal failure • Hemodynamic Instability • Respiratory failure • Large-volume ascites • Encephalopathy	ICU

(BUN: blood urea nitrogen; ICP: intracranial pressure; ISGLS: International Study Group of Liver Surgery; PHLF: posthepatectomy liver failure; UOP: urine output)

- >50% liver volume resected
- Major hepatectomy including right lobectomy
- Skeletonization of hepatoduodenal ligament
- <25% of liver volume remaining

Postoperative Management Associated
- Postoperative hemorrhage
- Intra-abdominal infection

Bile Leakage after Hepatobiliary and Pancreatic Surgery

ISGLS Definition and Grading of Bile Leakage after Hepatobiliary and Pancreatic Surgery

Bile leakage is defined as fluid with an increased bilirubin concentration in the abdominal drain or in the intra-abdominal fluid on or after postoperative day 3, or as the need for radiologic intervention (i.e., interventional drainage) because of biliary collections or relaparotomy resulting from bile peritonitis. Increased bilirubin concentration in the drain or intra-abdominal fluid is defined as a bilirubin concentration at least 3 times greater than the serum bilirubin concentration measured at the same time **(Table 3)**.[3]

After hepaticojejunostomy (HJ) in hepatobiliary surgery, causes of bile in drain in early postoperative period:
- So it can be technical fault or missed duct
- So go in for surgery, as <48 hours, we can try for repair.
- If beyond that, then tissue is unhealthy, so manage conservatively. Do USG, make it a controlled external biliary fistula (EBF). Can refeed bile if clear and culture negative.
- After 7–10 days if no decrease in output, plan percutaneous transhepatic biliary drainage (PTBD). Once output down, get magnetic resonance cholangiopancreatography (MRCP) done, rule out missed ducts. If missed ducts, then go in for surgery only after 6 weeks [bile duct injury (BDI) repair principles].
- If no missed ducts, follow-up the HJ with USG and liver function tests (LFTs), and grade as per McDonald criteria.
- If strictured HJ, do PTBD dilatation or revision HJ if failed PTBD dilatation.

TABLE 3: ISGLS grading of bile leakage after hepatobiliary and pancreatic surgery[3]

Grade	Management
Grade A	Bile leakage requiring no or little change in patients' clinical management
Grade B	Bile leakage requiring a change in patients clinical management (e.g., additional diagnostic or interventional procedures) but manageable without relaparotomy, or a Grade A bile leakage lasting for >1 week
Grade C	Bile leakage requiring relaparotomy

POST-PANCREATIC RESECTION COMPLICATIONS

Delayed Gastric Emptying
- Incidence: 6–50%
- Defined by ISGPS (International Study Group of Pancreatic Surgery)

ISGPS Definition of Delayed Gastric Emptying (DGE) (Table 4)[4]

TABLE 4: Consensus definition of DGE after pancreatic surgery				
DGE grade	NGT required	Unable to tolerate solid oral intake by POD	Vomiting/Gastric distention	Use of prokinetics
A	4–7 days or reinsertion > POD 3	7	±	±
B	8–14 days or reinsertion > POD 7	14	+	+
C	>14 days or reinsertion > POD 14	21	+	+

Note: To exclude mechanical causes of abnormal gastric emptying, the patency of either the gastrojejunostomy or the duodenojejunostomy should be confirmed by endoscopy or upper gastrointestinal gastrograph in series.

(DGE: delayed gastric emptying; NGT: nasogastric tube; POD: postoperative day)

Source: Wente MN, Bassi C, Dervenis C, et al. Delayed gastric emptying after pancreatic surgery: A suggested definition by the International Study Group of Pancreatic Surgery. Surgery. 2007;142:761.

Postoperative Pancreatic Fistula

ISGPS Definition of Postoperative Pancreatic Fistula (POPF)[5]

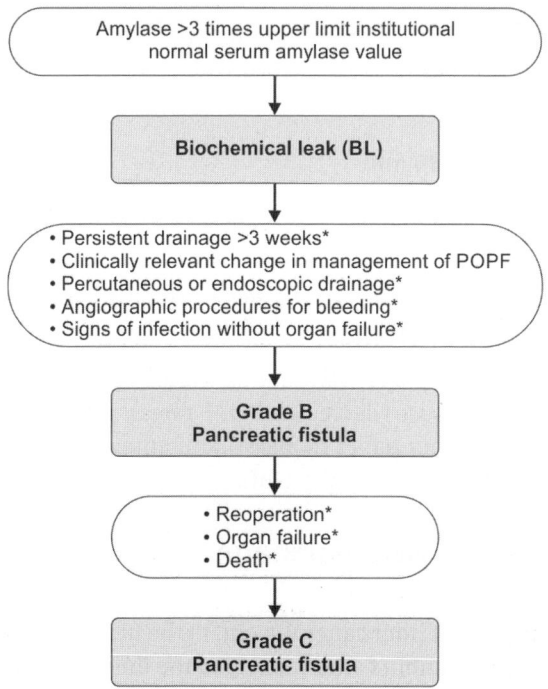

*Treatment/Event POPF related.

Fistula Risk Score Callery (Table 5)[6]

TABLE 5: Fistula risk score by Callery

Risk factor	Parameter	Points
Gland texture	Firm	0
	Soft	2
Pathology	Pancreatic adenocarcinoma or pancreatitis	0
	Ampullary, duodenal, cystic, islet cell	1
Pancreatic duct diameter (mm)	≥5	0
	4	1
	3	2
	2	3
	≤1	4
Intraoperative blood loss (mL)	≤400	0
	401–700	1
	701–1,000	2
	>1,000	3

Fistula Risk Zones (Table 6)[7]

TABLE 6: Fistula risk zones by Callery

Fistula risk zones	Points
Negligible	0
Low	1–2
Intermediate	3–6
High	7–10

POPF risk factors after distal pancreatectomy (DP):
- BMI >25
- Pancreatic thickness >15 mm
- Combined splenectomy
- Blood loss >1 L
- Prolonged surgery

No importance of texture and duct diameter (which are the principal elements of FRS leading to POPF after Whipple).

Techniques for closing stump after DP: Manual suture, falciform ligament, stapler, mesh, stapler + mesh closure (decreases POPF rates), glue, PJ (least POPF rates but higher morbidity, as per paper by Bassi) and antegrade PD stent (to reduce ductal pressure due to Oddi, but not useful).

Postpancreatectomy Hemorrhage

Time of onset:
- Early hemorrhage (≤24 hours after the end of the index operation)
- Late hemorrhage (>24 hours after the end of the index operation)

Location:
- Intraluminal (intranenteric, e.g., anastomotic suture line at stomach or duodenum, or pancreatic surface at anastomosis, stress ulcer, pseudoaneurysm)
- Extraluminal (extranenteric, bleeding into the abdominal cavity, e.g., from arterial or venous vessels, diffuse bleeding from resection area, anastomosis suture lines, pseudoaneurysm)

Severity of Hemorrhage

Mild:
- Small or medium volume blood loss (from drains, nasogastric tube, or on ultrasonography, decrease in hemoglobin concentration <3 g/dL)
- Mild clinical impairment of the patient, no therapeutic consequence, or at most the need for noninvasive treatment with volume resuscitation or blood transfusions (2–3 units packed cells within 24 hours of end of operation or 1–3 units if later than 24 hours after operation)
- No need for reoperation or interventional angiographic embolization; endoscopic treatment of anastomotic bleeding may occur provided the other conditions apply

Severe:
- Large volume blood loss (drop of hemoglobin level by ≥3 g/dL)
- Clinically significant impairment (e.g., tachycardia, hypotension, oliguria, hypovolemic shock), need for blood transfusion (>3 units packed cells)
- Need for invasive treatment (interventional angiographic embolization, or relaparotomy)

ISGPS Definition, Grading, Diagnostic and Therapeutic Consequences System of PPH (Table 7)[7]

Grade	Time of onset, location, severity and clinical impact of bleeding	Clinical condition	Diagnostic consequence	Therapeutic consequence
A	Early, intra- or extraluminal, mild	Well	Observation, blood count, ultrasonography and, if necessary, computed tomography	No
B	• Early, intra- or extraluminal, severe • Late, intra- or extraluminal, mild*	Often well/intermediate, very rarely life-threatening	Observation, blood count, ultrasonography, computed tomography, angiography, endoscopy	Transfusion of fluid/blood, intermediate care unit (or ICU), therapeutic endoscopy,[†] embolization, relaparotomy for early PPH

Continued

Continued

Grade	Time of onset, location, severity and clinical impact of bleeding	Clinical condition	Diagnostic consequence	Therapeutic consequence
C	Late, intra- or extraluminal, severe	Severely impaired, life-threatening	Angiography, computed tomography, endoscopy	Localization of bleeding, angiography and embolization, (endoscopy) or relaparotomy, ICU

* Late, intra- or extraluminal, mild bleeding may not be immediately life-threatening to patient but may be a warning sign for later severe hemorrhage ("sentinel bleed") and is therefore Grade B.
† Endoscopy should be performed when signs of intraluminal bleeding are present (melena, hematemesis, or blood loss via nasogastric tube).
(ICU: intensive care unit; PPH: postpancreatectomy hemorrhage)

Chyle Leak

ISGPS Definition and Grading System of Chyle Leak after Pancreatic Resection (Table 8)[8]

TABLE 8: Chyle leak grades and management

CL is defined as the output of milky-colored fluid from a drain, drain site, or wound, on or after postoperative day 3, with a triglyceride content ≥110 mg/dL or ≥1.2 mmol/L.

	Grade A	Grade B	Grade C
Therapeutic consequence	None or oral dietary restrictions*	Naso-enteral nutrition with dietary restriction* and/or TPN, percutaneous drainage by IR, maintenance of surgical drains, or drug (e.g., octreotide) treatment	Other invasive in-hospital treatment£, admission to the intensive care unit, and/or mortality¥
Discharge with (surgical) drain or readmission¥	No	Possibly	Possibly
Prolonged hospital stay¥	No	Yes	Yes

* No-fat diet with/without medium-chain-triglyceride
£ Interventional radiology (excluding percutaneous drainage) or reoperation
¥ Related directly to the chyle leak
(IR: interventional radiology; TPN: total parenteral nutrition)

Postpancreatectomy Acute Pancreatitis (PPAP)[9]

ISGPS Definition and Grading of PPAP[9]

We defined PPAP as an acute inflammatory condition of the pancreatic remnant beginning within the first 3 postoperative days after a partial pancreatic resection. The diagnosis requires (1) a sustained postoperative serum hyperamylasemia (POH) greater than the institutional upper limit of normal for at least the first

48 hours postoperatively, (2) associated with clinically relevant features, and (3) radiologic alterations consistent with PPAP. Three different PPAP grades were defined based on the clinical impact: (1) grade postoperative hyperamylasemia, biochemical changes only; (2) grade B, mild or moderate complications; and (3) grade C, severe life-threatening complications.

Below is a routinely encountered preoperative procedure related complication apart from the ones mentioned above.

Post-ERCP Pancreatitis

Two definitions:
1. *Cottons criteria:*[10]
   - Mild (typical pain of AP, rise in amylase ≥3 times after 24 hours, with 3 days hospital stay)
   - Moderate (4–10 days hospital stay)
   - Severe (>10 days hospital stay/any intervention for necrosis)
2. *Revised Atlanta Classification definition:*[11]
   - Mild, moderate, and severe.

When amylase should be sent after ERCP?

Amylase in AP normally rises after 6–24 hours and peaks at 48 hours, and normalizes over 3–7 days.

Amylase is elevated in 75% after ERCP irrespective of symptoms. However, a normal amylase after 6 hours of ERCP has a high negative predictive value for pancreatitis, and hence can be done if discharge is planned after procedure.

■ REFERENCES

1. Rahbari NN, Garden OJ, Padbury R, Maddern G, Koch M, Hugh TJ, et al. Post-hepatectomy haemorrhage: a definition and grading by the International Study Group of Liver Surgery (ISGLS). HPB (Oxford). 2011;13(8):528-35.
2. Rahbari NN, Garden OJ, Padbury R, Brooke-Smith M, Crawford M, Adam R, et al. Posthepatectomy liver failure: a definition and grading by the International Study Group of Liver Surgery (ISGLS). Surgery. 2011;149(5):713-24.
3. Koch M, Garden OJ, Padbury R, Rahbari NN, Adam R, Capussotti L, et al. Bile leakage after hepatobiliary and pancreatic surgery: a definition and grading of severity by the International Study Group of Liver Surgery. Surgery. 2011;149(5):680-8.
4. Wente MN, Bassi C, Dervenis C, Fingerhut A, Gouma DJ, Izbicki JR, et al. Delayed gastric emptying (DGE) after pancreatic surgery: a suggested definition by the International Study Group of Pancreatic Surgery (ISGPS). Surgery. 2007;142(5):761-8.
5. Bassi C, Marchegiani G, Dervenis C, Sarr M, Hilal MA, Adham M, et al. The 2016 update of the International Study Group (ISGPS) definition and grading of postoperative pancreatic fistula: 11 years after. Surgery. 2017;161(3):584-91.
6. Callery MP, Pratt WB, Kent TS, Chaikof EL, Vollmer Jr CM. A prospectively validated clinical risk score accurately predicts pancreatic fistula after pancreatoduodenectomy. J Am Coll Surg. 2013;216(1):1-4.
7. Wente MN, Veit JA, Bassi C, Dervenis C, Fingerhut A, Gouma DJ, et al. Postpancreatectomy hemorrhage (PPH)–an international study group of pancreatic surgery (ISGPS) definition. Surgery. 2007;142(1):20-5.

8. Besselink MG, van Rijssen LB, Bassi C, Dervenis C, Montorsi M, Adham M, et al. Definition and classification of chyle leak after pancreatic operation: a consensus statement by the International Study Group on Pancreatic Surgery. Surgery. 2017;161(2):365-72.
9. Marchegiani G, Barreto SG, Bannone E, Sarr M, Vollmer CM, Connor S, et al. Postpancreatectomy acute pancreatitis (PPAP): definition and grading from the International Study Group for Pancreatic Surgery (ISGPS). Ann Surg. 2022;275(4):663-72.
10. Cotton PB, Lehman G, Vennes J, Geenen JE, Russell RC, Meyers WC, et al. Endoscopic sphincterotomy complications and their management: an attempt at consensus. Gastrointest Endosc. 1991;37(3):383-93.
11. Foster BR, Jensen KK, Bakis G, Shaaban AM, Coakley FV. Revised Atlanta classification for acute pancreatitis: a pictorial essay. Radiographics. 2016;36(3):675-87.

CHAPTER 4

Bile Duct Injury

■ HISTORY

So then if patient has presented in postoperative period after laparoscopic cholecystectomy, first take history of:
- **Pre-surgery symptoms** like only pain (biliary colic) but with fever (cholecystitis), duration of pain and fever (longer signifies chronic cholecystitis), and with jaundice becomes cholangitis or history of gall stones pancreatitis, any USG/CECT/MRCP/ERCP with stenting done and the reason for surgery.
- **Surgery related:** Whether emergency/elective, lap or open, any blood transfusions given, any attempt at open, any drain put, how many hours it lasted, anything communicated to relatives, and after that was he shifted to ICU.

Was specimen shown, did it have stones, was it sent for histopathological examination (HPE).
- **Early postoperative:** Was patient comfortable and able to tolerate oral diet or any undue symptoms like pain, fever, jaundice, then color/nature/volume of drain and trend, any drain related tests done, then if it was removed or any new tube placed, any fever with chills during this time, any imaging/tube placement/ERCP done, any relaparotomy done (for sepsis/early repair), when was discharge taken with/without tube.
- **Late postoperative:** Whether readmitted, trend of drain output now, how many days later presented with jaundice. So early, intermittent and with pain, consider choledocholithiasis (CDL), early and progressive consider clipped duct, late and progressive consider Benign biliary stricture (BBS)/missed gallbladder cancer (GBC) or perihilar cholangiocarcinoma (pHCC). Also, pruritus, clay colored stools (complete) versus cholic stools (partial obstruction or internal fistula), any associated pain/fever/vomiting/hematemesis, history of fat soluble vitamin deficiency and chronic liver disease (CLD), any loss of weight/appetite, any further treatment taken/given after coming here.

Then rapidly think about two possible situations of how the patient may present, and how you will manage (situations A and B):

Situation A

Just remember that if after laparoscopic cholecystectomy, any patient presents in early postoperative period with pain, abdominal distention, fever, sepsis, peritonitis OR bilious drain, then it is biloma (with its complications) or external biliary fistula (EBF) respectively due to any of the following reasons:
- Retained stone in common bile duct (CBD) causing cystic duct stump blowout
- Bile leak from gallbladder fossa from ducts of Luschka
- *Bile duct injury (BDI) with bile leak*: Cholangitis may also be present along with all these
- Bowel injury (however, thermal injury generally presents 1–2 weeks later)
    - Mostly duodenal (bilious contents)
    - Can be colonic (feculent contents)

So in exam, when giving a diagnosis after history, say post-laparoscopic cholecystectomy BDI or bowel injury, with a suspected biloma or controlled/uncontrolled EBF.

How to differentiate between BDI and bowel (duodenal) injury:
- *Drain/Pigtail/Percutaneous drain (PCD) amylase and bilirubin*: So in BDI only bilirubin is elevated whereas in bowel injury, both are elevated. Send cultures (always send ABC—amylase, bilirubin, cultures)
- *Skin excoriation seen if it is bowel injury*
- *Oral diet coming into drain in bowel injury*
- *Oral methylene blue stains drain fluid blue in bowel injury*
- *Colon injury may lead to feculent output in drain*

Strasberg classification of BDI:
- *Type A*: Cystic duct stump leak/ducts of Luschka leak
- *Type B*: Ligation of right posterior sectoral duct (no bile leak)
- *Type C*: Bile leak from a divided right posterior sectoral duct (bile leak seen)
- *Type D*: Lateral BDI [common hepatic duct (CHD)/CBD]
- *Type E*: Bile duct strictures resulting from bile duct transection (as classified by Bismuth). Complete transection in acute phase:
    - *E1*: Stricture in CHD > 2 cm away from hilum
    - *E2*: Stricture within 2 cm from the hilum
    - *E3*: Stricture at the hilum; however communication between right and left duct is maintained:
        – 3a floor intact
        – 3b floor disturbed, so from management point of view, similar to that of type 4
    - *E4*: Stricture at the hilum with separation of right and left ducts; i.e., communication between right and left duct is not maintained
    - *E5*: Combined stricture of aberrant sectoral duct and main bile duct

So two approaches to manage acute BDI with bile leak, for a patient referred to you:
1. *Aggressive approach (ENDOSCOPIC)*: First drain all collections, do USG to confirm the same, followed by early MRCP (to see retained CBD stone/type A or D injury). So if retained stone, then go for therapeutic ERCP with stone removal and stenting, and if type A or D injury, then go for therapeutic ERCP with stenting.
   If type B, C, or E on MRCP, then go for delayed repair.
2. *Conservative approach (preferred by SGPGI group)*: First drain all collections, convert uncontrolled to controlled EBF, confirm this with USG and even CECT if required.
   Then observe trend of drain output and then do delayed MR imaging with delayed repair.
   And if duodenal injury present, then manage with repair over T tube/tube duodenostomy and feeding jejunostomy (FJ).
   If colon injury, then manage with repair/resection and anastomosis (RA).

Situation B

When the patient presents only with jaundice +/- cholangitis post-laparoscopic cholecystectomy.

So it can be due to:
1. Retained stone (early) or choledochal cyst (+/- stones within)
2. Clipped/ligated duct (early)
   In both above cases, get USG and if no collections, get MRCP done, so if stone present then ERCP and removal, and if clipped duct present, then go in as soon as possible (ASAP) and remove the clip, then follow-up 6 monthly with LFTs and USG for any stricture development (maximum chance in first 3 years, but can be seen even upto 10 years).
   And if ligated duct, then if it is a favorable injury with dilated proximal ducts without any biliary sepsis and vascular injury, can go in for early repair.
3. Benign biliary stricture (BBS) (late jaundice) or even stump lithiasis causing Mirizzi's syndrome. BBS can be secondary to BDI, or it can be due to other causes like recurrent pyogenic cholangitis (RPC), primary sclerosing cholangitis (PSC), primary biliary cirrhosis (PBC), IgG4 cholangiopathy and even TB.
4. Missed GBC infiltrating CHD/CBD or perihilar cholangiocarcinoma (pHCC) (late jaundice), if suspected, then look for mass on MRI and even cholangioscopy and biopsy, and get CA 19-9 done.

So in the above situation in exam, say my diagnosis is: Status post-laparoscopic cholecystectomy with above mentioned DDs.

Coming back to the present, now how to proceed after history and examination: Ask to review previous records of tests and imaging: Preoperative thick walled GB (TWGB) can be acute/chronic cholecystitis or xanthogranulomatous cholecystitis (XGC) or even gallbladder cancer (GBC) if thickening is focal, irregular, non-uniform or if polypoidal lesion or mass is seen, OT notes (difficult GB/Calot's, any suspicion of GBC-adherent omentum, TWGB, any bleeding/injury, did he cut open and examine specimen), *And most importantly, ask for GB histopathological examination report (HPR) (? malignancy)*, and any postoperative imaging/ERCP. Speak to the primary surgeon if possible regarding these details and ask for video of surgery.

Then after initial hydration, first do USG and even CECT if required to rule out/drain bilomas and send it for ABC—amylase, bilirubin and culture/sensitivity (C/S). However, if drain is in place for more than 1 week then it is likely to be colonized, and no point in sending C/S, however, freshly aspirated collection can still be sent for C/S. Aim to convert any uncontrolled EBF to controlled.

Do complete hemogram, LFT, KFT, SE, PT INR.

Then as per your approach: Aggressive or conservative, proceed accordingly as discussed above.

Remember that only after draining all collections, MRI, MRCP, MR angiogram (MRA) can be done. (Tubogram can be done as it is cheap, at least 2 weeks postinjury so that fistula tract has matured, but its fallacy is that it won't show disconnected biliary systems).

Professor VK Kapoor and Professor Sadiq Sikora have worked extensively on BDI. The following section is inspired from their teachings.

So BDI repair timing and success rate:
- *On table*: Best time for repair (only if below mentioned conditions are fulfilled)
- *Early*: Within 2 weeks (but most studies <72 hours)
- *Intermediate*: 2–6 weeks (worst time for repair)
- *Delayed*: 6 weeks to 6 months (best time for repair). Preferably 6 weeks to 3 months is the best time for repair, as secondary biliary cirrhosis (SBC) may develop as early as after 3 months, and definitely after 6 months.

So best time for repair is on table (at which point injury has just occurred), provided only if:
- Expertise is available, along with good light and equipment—retractors, fine instruments and fine sutures
- There is a complete intraoperative cholangiogram available after the BDI
- It is a good Bismuth injury (type 1, 2, 3a—floor of confluence intact)
- There is no vascular injury (confirmed by Doppler), because if vascular injury is present, then collaterals at hilum take time to develop for the anastomosis to survive and heal.

If any of these is not fulfilled, then it is best to do a delayed repair.

So now in postoperative period, what all does MRI with MRCP and MRA show (to be done only after all efforts have been made to drain all the collections):
- T2 MRI shows any undrained collections, intrahepatic biliary radical dilatation (IHBRD) (only central, or also extending to periphery), crowding of ducts (signifying atrophy and hence injury on that side) with elongated, spread out ducts on contralateral side (signifying hypertrophy) and signs of SBC if it is been more than 3 months of injury [irregular, nodular surface

of liver, collaterals, splenomegaly—if present, immediately ask for upper gastrointestinal endoscopy (UGIE)]. Also if number of applied clips are >8, then there is a high chance of complex BDI (as per Musa's criteria)
- MRCP (from top of image to down), and multiple MRCP images to be seen before commenting. The worst image, injury-wise, is the one which shows the actual injury.

    So MRCP shows IHBRD, crowding of ducts signifying atrophy on that side with compensatory hypertrophy on contralateral side evidenced by longer and spread out ducts on that side, site and level of injury, any segment loss, any loop of jejunum close to the CHD signifying internal fistula, and any undrained collections appearing hyperintense.
- MRA shows vascular injury, and signs of SBC like venous collaterals, perigastric and perisplenic varices

Indications for doing early MRI with MRCP:
- To delineate collections (similar role as CECT, if CECT is contraindicated) to plan for percutaneuous drain placement (PCD).
- If patient has presented with early bile leak, then for aggressive approach as described above (after draining all collections):
  ○ To see stones/bilioenteric continuity if it is there (only after all collections are drained/controlled EBF). Even hepatobiliary scintigraphy (with HIDA/DISIDA/PIPIDA) can be used for the same purpose, but if there is a big EBF, then it may not show bilioenteric continuity even if it is there, as it preferentially flows out via the fistula (falsely negative).
  ○ So if stones present, then ERCP with stone removal and stenting to be done. If continuity is present, seen in type A and D injuries, then can consider early therapeutic ERCP with stenting. Generally as bile leak stops, stent can be removed as early as 2 weeks. However, if plan is to manage endoscopically only, then ≥3 stents are placed side by side and changed every 3 months, for up to 12 months, to prevent formation of stricture. However stricture can occur even after 10 years, so definitive endoscopic management may not always be effective, hence surgery should always be considered in good PS patients.
- If patient presents with early jaundice, then if MRCP shows clipped duct with maintained continuity, i.e., without transection, then can go in early to remove the clip, as described above.
- And if early repair is planned, then to have a complete cholangiogram before surgery (to be combined with MRA to rule out vascular injury precluding early repair)

Indications for including MRA also:
- If early repair is planned, as vascular injury precludes early repair as collaterals have not developed between right hepatic artery (RHA) and left hepatic artery (LHA) and anastomosis may leak and stricture.
- A complex biliovascular injury, with injury to right portal vein may also necessitate right hepatectomy in the immediate/early period due to necrosis of right liver.

- For all other repairs also, get MRA done, because if there is a major vascular injury combined with a high Bismuth type 3b (floor involved), or 4 or 5 injury, then right hepatectomy may have to be done.
- Also for medicolegal purpose.

Cases in which early repair can be considered:
- Laparoscopic cholecystectomy with completely ligated duct (after transection), good Bismuth type sparing the floor of the confluence (types 1, 2, 3a), dilated proximal ducts (secondary to clipping) and rapidly rising bilirubin with no bile leak/biloma, no biliary sepsis, no peritonitis and finally, no vascular injury (confirmed by Doppler).
- For all other cases, delayed repair has best results.

So approach and preparations when patient of BDI is being planned for surgery:

PART A: **Optimize patient, know the biopsy of GB**
- Hydration for jaundice and related renal dysfunction
- Complete control of sepsis by drainage of collections, control of cholangitis with bile culture specific antibiotics
- Vitamins A, D, E, K supplementation.
- Bile refeeding (only if clear, and culture is sterile), as bile loss causes dehydration, hyponatremia, hypokalemia, metabolic acidosis, endotoxemia, malabsorption, fat soluble vitamin deficiency. So all this can be prevented/corrected.
- Supervised nutritional rehabilitation with high calorie and protein diet.
- *Demand biopsy of gallbladder.*

PART B: **Rule out SBC before doing expensive MRI, then do MRI to rule out any missed cancer and to define injury for planning surgery**
- If patient has presented few months later as BBS, then clinical exam to look for signs of secondary biliary cirrhosis (SBC) (which can be seen as early as 3 months) like palpable nodular liver, palpable spleen along with complete baseline investigations (BLI), especially LFT to look for signs of chronic liver disease (CLD) like high bilirubin, low albumin, Albumin-Globulin reversal (AG reversal) and raised PT INR, then calculate Child's score and then USG abdomen and Doppler to look for altered liver echotexture, venous collaterals, ascites, splenomegaly and fibroscan to rule out cirrhosis, and then UGIE to look for varices. If SBC present, *then refer for transplant.*
- Then a complete good quality MRI, with MRCP and MRA for the above reasons, and also to look at liver surface, IHBRD, crowding of ducts signifying atrophy/hypertrophy complex (AHC), any cholangiolytic abscesses, ductal anatomy, *look for any associated mass lesion and try to get tissue diagnosis: if cancer present then plan accordingly,* any stones/strictures present and level of injury, segment loss, any loop of small bowel close to the biliary system signifying internal fistula, any stent seen inside, any collaterals/signal voids signifying vascular injury on MRA.

***PART C:* Get ready for hepatectomy with preoperative biliary drainage (PBD)/ difficult repair with percutaneous transhepatic biliary catheters (PTBC) and vitamin K before surgery**
- In case of uncontrolled cholangitis or situations where a right hepatectomy is anticipated, like: type 4/high biliovascular injury, with atrophy-hypertrophy complex present/multiple intrahepatic strictures with recurrent episodes of cholangitis, or in a high/complex injury repair presenting with stricture, or when it's a missed cholangiocarcinoma, then preoperative biliary drainage (PBD) must be done.
- For an anticipated difficult reconstruction—bad type 3, or type 4 or type 5 injury, PTBC should be placed for guiding intraoperative recognition of bile ducts by injecting methylene blue, saline or by intraoperative USG to look for the PTBCs, which can be used as transanastomotic stents, which are retained at least for 1 year.
- Remember to give injection vitamin K 10 mg IV OD preoperative for 5 days (even if INR is normal)

How to proceed during surgery:
Don't disturb the drain/PCD.

Right subcostal/J shaped/bilateral subcostal incision. Meticulous dissection from the start, be careful not to cut the liver while opening the muscle layer. Put Allis on the muscle layers and pull it up, while doing adhesiolysis between liver and abdominal wall. Then start from the right of the abdomen and proceed to the left. From the right, take down the hepatic flexure, duodenum, use the PCD to guide you to the BDI site, or if any internal fistula present, and leave it there till the end. Then proceed to hepatoduodenal ligament (HDL). *Palpate common hepatic artery (CHA) and proper hepatic artery (PHA)*, as CBD will be lateral to the pulsations. (Be wary of AHC in BDI cases as portal vein then could be anterior due to rotation. Hence confirm if bile present by aspirating with a fine needle before doing anything drastic). Lower the hilar plate by the Hepp–Couinaud approach, as the horizontal extrahepatic part of left hepatic duct (LHD) lies at the base of segment 4B.

How to identify ducts intraoperatively:
- Keep drain/PCD in place, it will guide you
- In case of an internal fistula, keep it till the end, use it as a guide
- Lowering of the hilar plate, exposing the hilum and horizontal part of left hepatic duct (if even now LHD is not found, then coring of base of segment 4B will expose LHD), then trace it to the right, lower the cystic plate as well, to find right sided ducts.
- Use of pre-/intraoperative placed PTBC by injecting saline, methylene blue
- Use of intraoperative USG and look for PTBC.
- If right sided ducts are not seen, then hepatotomy in GB fossa bed to expose right anterior sectoral duct, and then dissection around it to reach the confluence/right posterior sectoral duct (RPSD).

- Hepatotomy around Rouviere's sulcus to expose RPSD and then dissection around it to reach the confluence/right anterior sectoral duct (RASD).
- Use of on table ICG cholangiography (needs 30 minutes to 1 hour for dye to be excreted in ducts)
- If still unable to find duct, plan for hepatectomy.

Hepaticojejunostomy (HJ) stoma should be ideally 3 cm, as it shrinks to 1/3. Blumgart Kelly technique may be used (anterior sutures are preplaced, going from outside of jejunum so that final knot lies on outside, then posterior layer is completed, and finally anteriorly preplaced sutures are tied). However, at our place, we do the posterior layer first, followed by the anterior layer, with 4-0 vicryl (cheaper with easier knotting).

Also, dont forget to take liver biopsy to document fibrosis/base line liver status.

Follow-up of BDI repair: 3-6 monthly clinical examination for features of jaundice, pruritus, cholangitis and liver function tests (LFTs) for obstructive jaundice (OJ) and cholangitis, and USG abdomen for IHBRD, and if present, then magnetic resonance cholangiography (MRC).

Then grade as per McDonald/Mayo criteria:
- *A (Excellent)*: Normal LFT, no symptoms.
- *B (Good)*: Deranged LFT, no symptoms.
- *C (Fair)*: Deranged LFT and cholangitis.
- *D (Poor)*: Requires endoscopic/surgical intervention.

Practically speaking, only grades A and B are considered to be successful repairs.

Life-long follow-up is needed as delayed strictures can form and are most commonly seen in the first 2 years.

Management of postoperative HJ stricture:
- PTBD with balloon dilatation is the treatment of choice as it can help avoid re-do surgery.
- However, if not possible/persistent stricture despite multiple sessions of PTBD and balloon dilatation, then re-do surgery is the only option:
  - If proximal/left sided duct available, re-do HJ with wide stoma (as per the principles of a good HJ) can be done. If already a high repair was done previously or if the injury was complex (bad Bismuth type/associated with a vascular injury), then re-do HJ has poor results. Right hepatectomy may have to be done in this case, after doing preoperative biliary drainage (PBD) of left lobe.
- If features of SBC are present, then the only option which remains, is liver transplant.

CHAPTER 5

Chronic Pancreatitis

■ HISTORY AND EXAMINATION

History of abdominal pain: Pancreatitis related pain is dull aching, episodic, epigastric, radiating to back, and often precipitated/worsened by a fatty meal and relieved on bending forwards.

Increase in intensity of pain/worsening of pain (not getting relieved on oral medications but is requiring IV medication/opioids), forms an indication for surgery. Interference with academics or job also suggests need for intervention and recent change in nature of pain becoming continuous from intermittent, points toward malignant change.

History of persistence/recurrence of pain or upper abdominal lump points toward pseudocyst. However, mass arising on the background of chronic pancreatitis or palpable GB due to distal obstruction secondary to inflammatory biliary stricture/mass in head of pancreas (HOP) or splenomegaly secondary to sinistral portal hypertension (PHTN) can all be palpable and thus become differentials for lump in a case of chronic pancreatitis.

History of vomiting: In the setting of chronic pancreatitis, history of postprandial fullness and/or postprandial vomiting of gastric contents points toward gastric outlet obstruction (GOO) secondary to compression on the stomach, the differentials of which, in patients with chronic pancreatitis are:
- Pseudocyst
- Inflammatory/malignant head mass
- Inflammatory narrowing of duodenum

GI bleed: May occur due to either hemosuccus pancreaticus or left sided portal hypertension. Hemosuccus pancreaticus occurs due to pancreatic enzymes acting on the peripancreatic vessels resulting in pseudoaneurysm formation, which bleeds into the gastrointestinal (GI) tract via the pancreatic duct. Pancreatitis may result in splenic vein thrombosis which may lead to left sided portal hypertension with subsequent variceal bleed. Also grade the severity of bleed.

History of pruritus, yellowish discoloration of eyes, high colored urine, clay colored stools: Points toward obstructive jaundice, secondary to compression of CBD, the differentials of which, in patients with chronic pancreatitis are:
- Inflammatory edema of the acute (on chronic) attack
- Pseudocyst
- Benign biliary stricture (BBS)
- Inflammatory/malignant head mass

History of fever: As a part of systemic inflammatory response syndrome, or in case of infected pseudocyst or cholangitis.

History of steatorrhea: Exocrine insufficiency manifests in the form of steatorrhea, i.e., malabsorption of fats resulting in excessive loss of fats in stools (>7 g/day), which leads to oily, frothy, malodorous stools which are difficult to flush. Ask if the patient has been taking any tablets for the same (PERT) and if the steatorrhea has reduced/resolved

History suggestive of fat-soluble vitamin deficiency: Due to long term fat malabsorption. Night blindness (vitamin A), osteomalacia leading to fractures (vitamin D), male infertility (vitamin E) and hemorrhage (vitamin K).

History of diabetes mellitus: Endocrine insufficiency as one of the tripods of symptomatology of chronic pancreatitis manifests in the form of diabetes mellitus. However, remember that worsening of glycemic control is a harbinger of malignancy.

Weight loss is seen in chronic pancreatitis due to severe pain often leading to fear of consuming food, exocrine insufficiency and the resulting malabsorption. However, loss of weight combined with loss of appetite points toward malignant change.

Treatment history for established chronic pancreatitis:
- Multiple episodes of admission for IV analgesics/opioids suggest poor pain control and becomes an indication for surgery in chronic pancreatitis.
- *History of endoscopic procedure*: Done for pseudocyst (endoscopic cystogastrostomy), biliary obstruction (ERCP with biliary stenting) and pancreatic duct stones (ESWL followed by pancreatic duct stenting). Failure of endoscopic procedures again becomes an indication for surgery in chronic pancreatitis.

Treatment history for acute/recurrent acute pancreatitis:
- *History of ICU admission*: Points toward severe course of disease: SIRS, infected pancreatic necrosis, GI bleed.

Treatment history for infected pancreatic necrosis as a part of step up approach:
- *History of endoscopic procedure alone*: Endoscopic cystogastrostomy for pseudocyst (symptomatic/infected) or direct endoscopic necrosectomy for Walled off pancreatic necrosis (symptomatic/infected)

OR
- *History of percutaneous catheter drainage followed by minimally invasive surgery*: Video-assisted retroperitoneal debridement (VARD) or minimally

invasive retroperitoneal necrosectomy (MIRN) if not settling with PCD alone, followed by abdominal laparoscopic approach or eventually open approach, if not settling with minimally invasive retroperitoneal approaches.

History of surgery: Surgery in an emergency setting is done for:
- Abdominal compartment syndrome
- Bleeding causing hemodynamic instability [not managed by interventional radiology (IR)]
- Bowel ischemia
- Infected pancreatic necrosis or pancreatic hemorrhage with hemodynamic instability.

Past history of:
- Blunt abdominal trauma
- Biliary colic/cholecystectomy
- Painful bones, renal stones, psychic moans (hyperparathyroidism leading to chronic pancreatitis)
- COPD, infertility (cystic fibrosis-*CFTR* gene mutation leading to chronic pancreatitis)

Personal history of alcohol consumption and smoking (etiology for chronic pancreatitis).

Family history of pancreatitis is related to PRSS1, SPINK-1 and CFTR gene mutations.

■ EXAMINATION PROFORMA

General Examination: Part A
- *Visual appearance*:
  - Young/middle aged/elderly
- *Gender*:
  - Male/female
- *Built*: Poor/average/good
- *Nourishment:* Poor/average/good
  - Measure height, weight, BMI
- *Clinical evaluation*:
  - Conscious/stuporous
  - Cooperative/uncooperative
  - Orientation to time, place and person: Present/absent
  - Hydration status: Hydrated/dehydrated
  - Lying comfortably bed/in discomfort/in pain
  - Whether patient prefers sitting or lying down position
  - Febrile/Afebrile
  - Vitals: Pulse, BP, respiratory rate, mention performance status here as well

General Examination: Part B
Look for PICCLE, Oral Cavity, Skin
- PICCLE: Pallor, icterus, cyanosis, clubbing, generalized or localized lymphadenopathy, palpable cervical and left supraclavicular lymph node, pedal or dependent edema.
- Examination of oral cavity for hygiene, caries, mucosal lesions.
- Examination of skin for scratch marks (itching results due to obstructive jaundice).

Abdominal Examination
On inspection: See if—
- Any percutaneous drain (PCD) is in place (done for infected pancreatic necrosis)
- Note the nature of effluent: Serous/serosanguinous/sanguineous/purulent/seropurulent/milky (chylous) or cola colored (pancreatic fistula). Infected pancreatic necrosis has a dirty black/brown look
- Abdominal contour: Flat/distended/scaphoid
- Umbilicus: Central/displaced. Inverted/everted/flat
- All quadrants are moving equally with respiration or not

Look for any visible lump: Differentials of lump in abdomen in the context of chronic pancreatitis:
- Pseudocyst
- Inflammatory/malignant HOP mass
- Palpable GB secondary to distal CBD compression/block due to any of the above or benign biliary stricture (BBS)
- Palpable splenomegaly secondary to sinistral PHTN

If visible describe size, site, shape, surface and movement with respiration

- Look for scars of previous surgery or drain tube placement.
- Look for visible sinus, engorged veins, pulsations, peristalsis or cough impulse.
- Inspect the groin hernial sites and examine genitalia.
- Inspection of renal angles to look for fullness

On palpation: See if—
- Abdomen is soft, nontender

Remember the differentials of lump in abdomen in the context of chronic pancreatitis:
- Pseudocyst
- Inflammatory/malignant HOP mass
- Palpable GB secondary to distal CBD compression/block due to any of the above or BBS
- Palpable splenomegaly secondary to sinistral PHTN

If present describe:
- Site
- Size

- Shape
- Surface
- Margins
- Tenderness
- Consistency
- Mobility
- Movement with respiration
- *Plane*:
    - To help differentiate between abdominal wall and intra-abdominal masses, perform the leg raising test (also known as Carnett's test): a parietal mass will become more prominent while the patient raises their legs, while an intra-abdominal mass will become less prominent.
    - To help differentiate between intraperitoneal and retroperitoneal masses, perform the lateral decubitus test: A retroperitoneal mass will not fall ahead, while an intraperitoneal mass will.
- Palpate groin hernia sites and examine genitals
- Look for tenderness in renal angles
- Examine back and spine for tenderness.

On percussion:
- Look for upper border of liver dullness (generally in the 5th intercostal space) in midclavicular line.
- Note the liver span (normal being 12–14 cm)
- Percussion note over lump if any
- Percussion note over rest of the abdomen
- Tests for free fluid.

Differentials of the ascites in the context of chronic pancreatitis:
- Nutritional (hypoalbuminemia due to poor intake)
- Pancreatic (due to anterior pancreatic ductal disruption leading to pancreatic fistula communicating with the abdominal cavity)
- Malignant (head mass)

On auscultation:
- Auscultate for bowel sounds.
- Bruit, hum and rub
- *Per-rectal examination*: Look for metastatic deposits in the pouch of Douglas (Blumer Shelf)

Respiratory Examination

Increased tactile vocal fremitus on palpation, dull note on percussion and reduced breath sounds on auscultation are a clue toward pleural effusion (secondary to hypoalbuminemia or to posterior pancreatic ductal disruption forming a pancreatopleural fistula).

Rest systemic examination

■ RECURRENT ACUTE PANCREATITIS (RAP)[1,2]

Definition of recurrent acute pancreatitis (AP): At least >2 attacks of AP with at least 3 months gap in between, without any clinical or imaging features of chronic pancreatitis (CP).

Alcohol, gallstones, trauma (blunt, post-ERCP) are most common causes of AP and if not eliminated, can cause RAP. But 10–25% are idiopathic of which, the causes are listed below, which lead to RAP. However, even after all investigations, the cause would not be found for some, which are the truly idiopathic cases.

Idiopathic RAP is most commonly seen due to: Mechanical/anatomical or toxic metabolic or miscellaneous factors.

Mechanical and anatomical:
- *Microlithiasis*: <3 mm stones (diagnosis best with EUS ~96% sensitivity). *Treatment*: Cholecystectomy
- Biliary parasites
- *Pancreatobiliary tumors* (ampullary tumors and IPMNs present with RAP in ~5%): Best diagnosed with EUS
- Types 1 and 4 choledochal cyst (CDC)
- Type 3 CDC causing main pancreatic duct (MPD) obstruction: Treatment is endoscopic sphincterotomy
- *Sphincter of Oddi dysfunction (SOD)*: Type 1 SOD has best prognosis after sphincterotomy
- Pancreas divisum (PD) (only if associated with a second hit of genetic mutation like *CFTR, SPINK1, PRSS1*). In PD, majority pancreas drains through minor papilla (longer superior duct), while the lower duct is small, drains only lower part of head and uncinate into major papilla. So on MR, PD appears as crisscrossing of the pancreatic duct with the CBD, whereas, a normal pancreatic duct meets the CBD at the lower end.
  Treatment is minor papilla sphincterotomy.

Toxic metabolic:
- Hypercalcemia
- Hypertriglyceridemia
- Drugs

Miscellaneous:
- Vascular
- Hereditary, familial pancreatitis
- Early CP (presents without calcification and ductal dilatation in it's initial stages)

1st phase investigations after 1st attack of AP:
- *History and examination*: Alcohol, biliary colic, trauma, viral illness (measles, mumps, rubella), painful bones and renal stones for hyperparathyroidism, dry eyes and dry mouth for autoimmune pancreatitis (AIP), chest infections and infertility for cystic fibrosis (CF), then drugs and family history.

- *Biochemistry*: LFT (Bilirubin >3, ALT ≥3 times: means biliary pancreatitis. ALT >150 ~96% sensitive for it. Abnormal LFT in 48 hours, with a normal USG, suspect microlithiasis), calcium, lipids.
- *Imaging*: USG, CECT.

If negative, then labeled as idiopathic pancreatitis, and proceed to 2nd phase investigations.

2nd phase:
- EUS done 6–8 weeks of acute attack, so changes of AP resolve and CP if present can be diagnosed better.
    - EUS is best for diagnosis of microlithiasis, occult biliary tumors, congenital anomaly of the pancreas like divisum, early CP, evaluation of CP with head mass, and for evaluation of location of pseudocysts for possible drainage and for other cystic lesions for which EUS FNA can be done.
    - The changes suggestive of CP include both parenchymal (hyperechoic foci, hyperechoic strands, parenchymal lobularity, calcification) and ductal (pancreatic duct dilatation, irregularity, hyperechoic walls, visible side branches)
    - Rosemont major criteria: Hyperechoic foci with shadowing, lobularity with honeycombing, and MPD calculi.
- MRCP and Secretin MRCP if needed to rule out IPMN
- ERCP followed by bile microscopy to look for biliary crystals (indirect sign of microlithiasis), manometry (for suspected SOD)

If negative, then
3rd phase:
Genetic testing for *SPINK1*, *PRSS1*, *CFTR* (with sweat chloride test).

Just remember:
- AP, RAP and CP form a continuum
- Truly idiopathic RAP most often progresses to CP, hence regular follow-up recommended.
- Approximately 40–45% of RAP proceed to CP (necrosis-fibrosis and SAPE hypotheses).

■ TRIALS IN INFECTED NECROTIZING PANCREATITIS

1. PANTER: Step up approach: Percutaneous drainage (PCD) or endoscopic drainage followed by VARD/MIRP followed by open versus upfront open surgery. So 35% settled with PCD alone
2. PENGUIN (JAMA 2010): Endoscopic step up: Drainage followed by direct endoscopic necrosectomy (DEN)] versus upfront surgical. Death rates equal. Lesser perforation, pancreatic fistula (PF), new onset organ failure, endo and exocrine insufficiency, incisional hernia in endoscopic group
3. TENSION (LANCET 2017): Endoscopic step up versus surgical. PF and length of stay (LOS) less in endoscopic group

4. MISER (J GASTRO 2019): Endoscopic step up versus minimally invasive surgery. None of the patients in endoscopic group had enteral or PF (vs. 28% in surgery) and physical quality of life (QOL) scores much better and cost lesser than compared to surgical.
5. POINTER (NEJM 2021): Immediate (≥24 hours of suspicion of infected necrosis) versus delayed PCD [after stage of Walled off necrosis (WON)]. So delayed PCD better as lesser complications and necrosectomy procedures required.

■ CHRONIC PANCREATITIS

Characterized by tripod of pain, exocrine pancreatic insufficiency (EPI) and endocrine insufficiency along with fibroinflammatory destruction of the pancreas.

EPI causes, diagnosis, management: Different causes of EPI in general: (DDs of EPI/steatorrhea can be asked during viva):
1. *Pancreatic causes*: Acute necrotizing pancreatitis, CP, and following pancreatic resectional surgeries
2. *Nonpancreatic causes*:
   - Celiac disease
   - Crohn disease
   - Zollinger–Ellison syndrome

EPI results in decreased absorption of:
- Fat including essential fatty acids
- Fat-soluble vitamins A, D, E and K
- Calcium, magnesium, zinc, thiamine and folic acid

Patients with EPI frequently experience:
- Abdominal distention, abdominal discomfort and/or pain, flatulence, diarrhea and grossly as steatorrhea [classically defined as at least 7 g of fecal fat over 24 hours (100 g of fat daily for 72 hours)] and weight loss
- Anemia resulting from malabsorption can be either microcytic (related to iron deficiency) or macrocytic (related to vitamin B12 deficiency).
- Intermediate and long-term malnutrition from EPI increases the incidence of osteopenia/osteoporosis, low-trauma fractures, cardiovascular diseases and infections.

The diagnostic options for EPI include:
- Indirect measures (i.e., 72-hour fecal fat and fecal elastase) or
- Direct measures (i.e., secretin–cerulein or secretin–pancreozymin tests).

Pancreatic Enzyme Replacement Therapy (PERT)
- Pancreatic enzymes are derived from swine or Ox pancreas
- Pancreatic enzyme products contains three pancreatic enzymes (i.e., amylase, protease, and lipase)
- Approximately 25,000–40,000 IU of lipase is required to digest a typical meal, and about 5,000–25,000 IU of lipase per snack.

- Enteric coated (EC)-bicarbonate-buffered PERT has previously been shown to produce a significant increase in fat absorption in cystic fibrosis (CF) patients compared with treatment with EC-nonbuffered PERT at equivalent lipase doses.
- Lipase doses >6,000 units/kg/meal are associated with colonic stricture (fibrosing colonopathy)

Monitoring therapy:
- *Clinical improvement*:
    - Weight gain
    - Symptomatic improvement in diarrhea
    - Degree of symptom improvement does not always correlate with the patient's nutritional status
- *Blood investigations*:
    - Serum retinol-binding protein, ferritin, and prealbumin
- *Carbon-13 breath test*: 13C-labeled mixed triglyceride breath test
- Coefficient of fecal fat absorption (CFA)

If no improvement, get fecal chymotrypsin levels done (if normal, then it is good compliance, if not, then counsel).

So if it's normal, then change diet: Fat maximum 50–75 g/day, low fiber, no alcohol, increase lipase dose, and add PPI or H2 blockers.

If still no results, then check for alternative causes (bacterial overgrowth, blind loop syndrome, other secondary causes of diarrhea).

Complications of CP
- Pseudocyst
- Complications of pseudocyst like causing GOO, bleeding into cyst which may present as hemosuccus pancreaticus, CBD obstruction and cholangitis, infection, rupture leading to pancreatic ascites/pleural effusion
- Inflammatory mass/cancer in HOP
- Duodenal stenosis/BBS
- Splenic vein thrombosis leading to left sided PHTN, splenomegaly and gastric varices causing UGI bleed
- Arterial pseudoaneurysms

Lump in a Case of CP May be Due to
- Pseudocyst
- Inflammatory mass/cancer in HOP itself
- Distended stomach due to GOO (secondary to pseudocyst, mass, duodenal stenosis)
- Distended GB due to distal BBS or secondary to lower CBD compression due to pseudocyst/inflammatory mass/cancer in HOP
- Splenomegaly secondary to left sided PHTN due to splenic vein thrombosis

Causes of Jaundice in CP
- Cholelithiasis (CL) with choledocholithiasis (CDL)
- Inflammatory edema of acute attack

- BBS
- Lower CBD compression due to pseudocyst/inflammatory mass/cancer in HOP

Clinical Pointers Toward Malignancy Developing in CP
- Change in the nature of pain, with episodic/intermittent becoming more continuous
- Progressively deepening jaundice
- Recent onset of DM (within 2 years of CP)/worsening of glycemic control OR onset after 50 years of age
- Anorexia with profound weight loss
- Tropical CP (non-alcoholic, young, large ductal stones) has more chances than alcoholic CP for malignancy

So now, to Begin with, Ask for Two Sets of Investigations for CP
One to confirm/arrive at a diagnosis and assess for complications and other to complete the workup of the patient.

So for workup:
- All blood tests
- *See LFT*: Raised bilirubin, ALP, GGT in OJ due to CDL/BBS or malignancy, also deranged LFT with enzymes seen in alcoholic hepatitis/cholangitis

And additionally:
- Serum amylase, lipase (to rule out acute on CP)
- Serum PTH level, calcium, lipids (as all can cause recurrent AP and lead to CP). Get IgG4 and sweat chloride test if indicated.
- For endocrine insufficiency: Blood glucose, HbA1c, glucose tolerance test (GTT)
- For exocrine insufficiency: Fecal fat, Sudan stain, fecal elastase (low levels <100 seen in CP) and fecal chymotrypsin (low levels seen when not compliant with PERT)
- *Ask for* Ca 19-9 for any suspicion of malignancy *only after USG abdomen and CXR* (to be repeated after biliary decompression)
- *For diagnosis*: USG to show status of liver (alcoholic), any space occupying lesion (SOL), IHBRD, status of GB (CL), CBD (CDL/BBS), pancreas for changes of CP like atrophy, calcifications, calculi, ductal dilatation, chain of lakes and complications of CP like pseudocyst, mass, ascites (nutritional or pancreatic or malignancy), pleural effusion, venous thrombosis, collaterals, varices, splenomegaly, pseudoaneurysms. Also look for peripancreatic fat stranding to rule out acute pancreatitis.
- Plain X-ray to see stones from L1 at right, to left of abdomen
- CECT to have a geographical location of stone load and to better assess other above-mentioned complications of CP as CECT is more sensitive than USG for all this and also to evaluate the mass.
- MRI abdomen for better delineation of any cystic lesion in pancreas or any indeterminate lesion in liver with MRCP for the ductal anatomy (CBD for CDL, BBS, and MPD for strictures, dilatations).

- UGIE to look for ulcers, varices, bulge of pseudocyst, side viewing endoscopy (SVE) to assess periampullary region.
- EUS which will help to know microlithiasis (<3 mm stones), early CP by Rosemont criteria, EUS guided cystogastro/enterostomy and direct endoscopic necrosectomy can be done.
- EUS-FNA may help to take biopsy from head mass (EUS FNA is more preferable for head mass than tail mass, as in latter it may lead to peritoneal seeding).
- EUS will also help characterize cystic lesions of pancreas, and EUS FNA of cyst fluid for analysis can be done.

So Four Objective Criteria for HOP Mass in CP to be Malignant: (Stanley Criteria)

1. Raised bilirubin (>5.8 mg/dL)
2. Raised CA19-9 (>127)
3. Dilated CBD (14.5 mm)
4. Dilated MPD (11.5 mm)

Other Objective Pointers of the HOP Mass Being Malignant

- Imaging features: Heterogeneously hypoenhancing in arterial phase on CECT (whereas inflammatory mass is homogeneously hyperenhancing), with diffusion restriction on DW-MRI, with high SUV max on FDG PET CT.
- Confirmation by EUS FNA.

Standard Indications of Surgery in CP

- Intractable pain (not relieved by conservative treatment or requiring frequent and/or persistent use of opiates, side effects of narcotics/addiction and/or interfering with QOL).
- Inflammatory complications:
  - Symptomatic pseudocyst causing GOO, UGI bleed (due to bleed within the cyst resulting in hemosuccus pancreaticus OR splenic vein thrombosis secondary to inflammation leading to left sided PHTN with gastric varices) or peritoneal bleeding due to ruptured pseudoaneurysm, symptomatic CBD obstruction (jaundice/cholangitis), infected cyst or rupture leading to pancreatic ascites or pleural effusion.
  - Inflammatory mass causing GOO/CBD obstruction
  - Duodenal stenosis causing GOO
  - BBS leading to symptomatic CBD obstruction
- HOP mass suspicious for cancer (Stanley criteria + imaging features of mass on CECT, DW-MRI and FDG PET CT + confirmation with EUS FNA)

ESCAPE Trial in CP

Early surgery ≤3 years of onset of pain leads to better pain control and QOL along with better preservation of pancreatic function.

Dilated CBD, with Dilated main Pancreatic Duct (MPD) in CP, Consider
- CDL
- CDC
- BBS
- Intraductal papillary mucinous neoplasm-Biliary (IPMN-B)
  All of the above cause dilated CBD, and may be seen with a dilated MPD due to CP itself or with an intraductal papillary mucinous neoplasm-Pancreatic (IPMN-P) associated also with CP.
- Periampullary lesion
- CP with head mass

Cause of Hugely Dilated CBD and Hugely Dilated MPD with Normal Bilirubin (So Nonobstructing Cause)
CDC/IPMN-B with CP/IPMN-P.

Causes of Hugely Dilated MPD with Normal Bilirubin
- CP
- IPMN-P

Types of Surgery for CP (Only the Ones in Actual Practice are Mentioned and Discussed Here)
- Drainage [lateral pancreaticojejunostomy (LPJ)]
- Resectional (DPPHR—Duodenum preserving pancreatic head resection—Beger's procedure and Whipple and total pancreatectomy)
- Hybrid procedures (Frey's and Izbicki) and
- For pain—celiac plexus block, thoracoscopic splanchnicectomy

Drainage Procedures
Lateral Pancreaticojejunostomy
Indication:
For ductal disease with dilated (>6 mm) pancreatic duct and pancreatic ductal calculi without inflammatory mass in the head/bulky head.

Crux of the procedure:
Pancreatic duct is filleted open along its entire length from the head to the tail, stones are removed and the opened duct is anastomosed side-to-side with a Roux-en-Y loop of jejunum. Extremely important to open the duct and remove the stones entirely in the tail, minor ducts and also in the uncinate region. *Not doing so* may lead to recurrent attacks of acute on chronic CP and pseudocyst formation which renders the index operation futile, thus giving LPJ a bad name.

How to identify the pancreatic duct:
- If the duct is dilated on imaging, then it may be seen obviously or felt as a fluctuant longitudinal bulge on the anterior surface of the body of the pancreas between its upper and lower borders

- Needle puncture on the anterior surface of the body of the pancreas midway between the superior and inferior borders and aspiration of clear watery pancreatic fluid or hitting a large stone with a gritty sensation transmitted while doing so
- Head coring of pancreatic parenchyma as is done in Freys
- Intraoperative ultrasound to locate the duct followed by USG guided needle puncture
- Duodenotomy and cannulation of the pancreatic ampullary orifice with an infant feeding tube
- Preoperative placement of pancreatic stent

Advantage:
?Preservation of pancreatic function.

Disadvantage:
Cannot drain ducts completely in a bulky head/inflammatory HOP mass which form the indications for performing a hybrid/resectional procedure.

Resectional Procedures

Beger

Indication: Inflammatory mass in the head of pancreas.

Crux of the procedure:
Resection of the pancreatic head anterior to the portal vein-small rim of pancreatic parenchyma within the C loop of duodenum is preserved to protect the pancreato-duodenal arcades and the duodenal blood supply. Pancreas is transected at its neck (in front of the superior mesenteric vein portal vein). The remaining pancreas (along C loop on one side and body on the other) is anastomosed to a Roux loop of jejunum. Two pancreaticojejunal anastomoses to the same Roux loop (one to the end of the distal pancreas and other to the rim of the pancreatic tissue in the head).

Advantage:
Relieves biliary obstruction as well (which is however, relieved even with a Frey's procedure which is much safer to perform as it avoids the dangerous dissection and division of the pancreatic neck in front of the portal vein).

Disadvantages:
- Risky due to above-mentioned reason.
- Loss of parenchyma more as compared to LPJ and Freys—Higher risk of exocrine (steatorrhea) and endocrine (diabetes) insufficiency.
- Does not address the pancreatic duct in the body and tail and hence, should not be performed as the sole procedure in such case.

Modifications:
Berne modification: Pancreas is not transected at its neck and the cored head is anastomosed to a Roux loop of jejunum—with only a single anastomosis.

Whipple

Indication:
HOP mass likely to be malignant as per stanley/other objective criteria mentioned above.

Advantage:
- R0 resection possible as tumor planes not breached as would be in head coring
- Relieves biliary obstruction as well
- Pacemaker of pain resected

Disadvantages:
- Loss of parenchyma more as compared to LPJ and Freys—Higher risk of exocrine (steatorrhea) and endocrine (diabetes) insufficiency
- Higher morbidity due to POPF/PPH/DGE

Total Pancreatectomy with Islet Auto-transplantation (IAT)

Indication:
Rescue surgery in intractable pain of chronic pancreatitis (after previous surgery for CP).

Requires:
Preserved islet cell function, which is a rarity due to endocrine insufficiency seen with CP.

Advantage:
When compared to Whipples procedure, in addition to its advantages, there is no morbidity of POPF as there is no pancreatic anastomosis.

Disadvantages:
- Brittle diabetes (insulin and glucagon, both are lost) and severe exocrine insufficiency (however, both are manageable medically)
- Autonomic sensitization may lead to pain even after such an extensive procedure

Hybrid Procedures: Drainage + Resection Combined

Frey's Procedure

Indication:
Bulky head/inflammatory HOP mass along with ductal strictures/stones in the pancreatic duct in body and tail.

Crux of the procedure: Head coring + LPJ
So unroofing of the pancreatic ducts in head and uncinate process of the pancreas anterior to the ducts or up to the posterior capsule+ opening of the entire pancreatic duct in the body and tail + LPJ.

Ligation of ASPDA branch of Gastro-duodenal artery (GDA) helps decrease bleeding during the coring of the head.

Also, bleeding due to injury to the anterior pancreaticoduodenal arcade of vessels between the head of the pancreas and the C loop of the duodenum can be prevented by taking multiple deep sutures in the pancreatic parenchyma 0.5–1 cm away from the pancreaticoduodenal groove.

Advantages:
- Helps to identify an undilated pancreatic duct
- Drains all ducts in the head and uncinate process (achieved with anterior coring)
- Removes pacemaker of the pain in CP, which is the head of the pancreas (achieved with posterior coring)
- A well performed Frey's even decompresses the obstructed CBD

Izbicki Procedure

Indication:
Undilated ducts in the parenchyma with diffuse stone disease.

Crux of the procedure:
Excision of a V-shaped wedge of the parenchyma anterior to the pancreatic duct to expose the undilated pancreatic duct, followed by jejunal anastomosis.

Hamburg modification – Izbicki procedure + head coring

Few Tips in Surgery for Chronic Pancreatitis (CP)

How is obstructed (dilated) CBD in CP handled?
- CBD may get decompressed by head coring alone in Frey's: pre and post-coring intraoperative cholangiogram (IOC) will confirm this
- CBD may get opened unintentionally into the cored out cavity in Frey's. So at that time it may be marsupialized–the walls of the opened CBD sutured to the pancreatic parenchyma to keep it open. But this has high stricture rates, so even in this situation, a formal choledochoduodenostomy (CDD) OR choledochojejunostomy (CDJ) in the same loop OR HJ in a separate loop, is preferred.
- CDD is an option if the duodenum is soft, supple and can be easily mobilized.
- CDJ may be done into the same Roux loop of the jejunum into which LPJ is done.
- HJ is the best (done to a separate loop of jejunum) as BBS in CP may often be long, extending proximally, which may lead to inadequate drainage with CDD/CDJ.
- Biliary diversion with CDD/CDJ/HJ alone, if pancreatic ductal surgery is not indicated (rare).

What all to be handled during surgery for CP:
1. Drainage of MPD, parenchyma and pseudocyst (in same loop)
2. In case of BBS, drainage of CBD (discussed above)
3. If left sided PHTN with varices, then add splenectomy

4. *If head mass/distal CBD stricture suspicious for malignancy, or even one EUS or intraoperative core biopsy (for head mass) or ERCP brush cytology/biopsy (of stricture) is suspicious for malignancy, then directly proceed with whipple/ Distal pancreatosplenectomy* (Depending upon where the mass is), and do additional procedures for CP as required as per points 1-3.
5. In a case of CP with pseudocysts, with a malignancy, if there has been an acute attack of pancreatitis get a MDT discussion.

Ideally wait for at least 4 weeks for inflammation to resolve, and in the mean time, do EUS guided cystogastrostomy and simultaneously start on NACT, and then re-stage and operate for malignancy, while also addressing the CP and pseudocysts (if was not addressed adequately endoscopically).

■ REFERENCES

1. Kedia S, Dhingra R, Garg PK. Recurrent acute pancreatitis: an approach to diagnosis and management. Trop Gastroenterol. 2013;34(3):123-35.
2. Machicado JD, Yadav D. Epidemiology of Recurrent Acute and Chronic Pancreatitis: Similarities and Differences. Dig Dis Sci. 2017;62(7):1683-91.

CHAPTER 6

Non-cirrhotic Portal Hypertension

■ HISTORY

History of vomiting blood (hematemesis): Spontaneous bleed is indicative of portal hypertensive bleed or peptic ulcer bleed or due to arteriovenous malformation (AVM)/Dieulafoy whereas hematemesis following retching is indicative of bleed due to Mallory Weiss tear.

Increased frequency of bleeding episodes, presence of blood clots is indicative of severe bleed and vomiting bright red/fresh blood is indicative of active bleed, whereas coffee ground vomitus is indicative of collected blood

Passage of melena: Seen in all cases of upper gastrointestinal (UGI) bleeding. However, hematochezia along with hematemesis is indicative of massive upper GI bleed or a second source of GI bleed in distal GI tract.

History of pain associated with hematemesis: Bleed due to AVM/Dieulafoys or varices is painless whereas due to peptic ulcer/Mallory Weiss due to retching is painful.

History of postural dizziness, syncope, fatigue, shortness of breath, requirement of hospitalization, need for blood transfusion and endoscopic treatment—To know the severity of blood loss.

Ascites, hepatic encephalopathy and jaundice all three individually or together point toward hepatic decompensation: Seen in cirrhotics even before bleeding and transiently in patients of non-cirrhotic portal fibrosis (NCPF) but only after an episode of bleeding. Remember that patients of extrahepatic portal venous obstruction (EHPVO) have bleeding episodes which are well tolerated. Also remember that NCPF patients can progress to cirrhosis, so the disease which was NCPH to begin with can very well culminate into cirrhosis.

History of lump in abdomen, left upper quadrant heaviness—indicative of splenomegaly.
- History of sudden onset left upper quadrant pain—indicative of splenic infarction
- History to suggest hypersplenism

- In 1955, Dameshek summarized that hypersplenism should be diagnosed in the presence of four conditions: (i) monolineage or mutilineage peripheral cytopenias; (ii) compensatory hyperplasia of bone marrow; (iii) splenomegaly; and (iv) correction of cytopenias after splenectomy.

Non-cirrhotic portal hypertension especially EHPVO may be associated with portal cavernoma cholangiopathy (PCC). Symptomatic PCC presents as jaundice and even as cholangitis.

Jaundice as a symptom in background of this disease process is indicative of either: Portal cavernoma cholangiopathy or hepatic decompensation

Fever is indicative of either: Systemic infections secondary to leukopenia resulting from hypersplenism or cholangitis (symptomatic PCC).

History of delayed achievement of milestones, growth retardation, delay in sexual development and poor scholastic performance: Seen with EHPVO.

Perinatal history: History of domiciliary birth and umbilical vein catheterization, umbilical sepsis, delayed separation of cord, abdominal sepsis secondary to appendicitis, pancreatitis, liver abscess—followed by surgery for the same: is indicative of abdominal infection during neonatal period or infancy which leads to portal venous thrombosis and is the etiology for NCPH (EHPVO > NCPF) as explained by the unifying hypothesis proposed by Kumar and Sarin in their seminal paper.

History of oral contraceptive (OC) pill consumption: Prothrombotic disposition.

History of spontaneous abortion: Indicative of antiphospholipid antibody syndrome.

History of alcohol abuse: Indicative of alcoholic liver disease and thus steers the diagnosis more toward cirrhosis *(do not marry your diagnosis, otherwise you will get divorced with your degree. Make an unemotional diagnosis after assessing all information).*

Prior history high-risk behavior, blood transfusion, recurring jaundice: Will again steer the diagnosis more toward viral hepatitis related cirrhosis.

Performance history: As per ECOG (Eastern Cooperative Oncology Group) classification to know if the patient will tolerate surgical stress. If not, then nonsurgical treatment options have to be relied upon.

■ EXAMINATION PROFORMA

General Examination: Part A
- *Visual appearance*:
  - Young/middle aged/elderly
- *Gender*:
  - Male/female
- *Built*: Poor/average/good
- *Nourishment:* Poor/average/good
  - Measure height, weight, BMI

- *Clinical evaluation*:
  - Conscious/stuporous
  - Cooperative/uncooperative
  - Orientation to time, place and person: Present/absent
  - Hydration status: Hydrated/dehydrated
  - Lying comfortably bed/in discomfort/in pain
  - Whether patient prefers sitting or lying down position
  - Febrile/Afebrile
- *Vitals*: Pulse, BP, respiratory rate, mention performance status here as well

General Examination: Part B

Look for PICCLE, oral cavity, skin, features of chronic liver disease (CLD):
- PICCLE: Pallor, icterus, cyanosis, clubbing, generalized or localized lymphadenopathy, palpable cervical and left supraclavicular lymph node, pedal or dependent edema
- *Sites to look for icterus*: Sclera/bulbar conjunctiva, undersurface of tongue, Soft palate, palms and soles.
- Skin for scratch marks secondary to pruritus (symptomatic PCC)
- *Stigmata of chronic liver disease (top to bottom):*
  - Icterus
  - Malar erythema
  - Fetor hepaticus
  - Parotid swelling
  - Spider nevi/spider angiomata
  - Gynecomastia
  - Reduced chest hair
  - Reduced axillary hair
  - Dupuytren contracture
  - Palmar erythema
  - Leukonychia
  - Flapping tremors/Asterixis
  - Abdominal distension
  - Caput medusae
  - Reduced pubic hair
  - Testicular atrophy
  - Pedal edema

Abdominal Examination

On Inspection: See if
- Abdominal contour: Flat/distended/scaphoid
- Umbilicus: Central/displaced. Inverted/everted/flat
- All quadrants are moving equally with respiration or not
- *Look for any visible lump*: Enlarged spleen

If visible describe:
- Size
- Site
- Shape
- Surface
- Movement with respiration (any organ with direct/indirect attachment to diaphragm, moves)

Look for dilated or engorged veins over the abdomen or flank:
- Dilated peri-umbilical veins radiating away from the umbilicus is indicative of portal hypertension.
- Dilated veins in craniocaudal orientation in the flank is indicative of caval obstruction

Look for visible scar, sinus, pulsations, peristalsis or cough impulse.

On palpation: See if
- Abdomen is soft and non-tender
- Liver is palpable or not
  If palpable, measure size from costal margin in midclavicular line in unit of cm or number of fingers,

See if:
- *It is tender/nontender:*
  ○ Surface is smooth (normal)/nodular (cirrhosis)
- Borders are round (fatty liver/ steatotic liver)/sharp (normal), regular (normal)/irregular (cirrhosis):
  ○ Consistency is soft (normal)/firm (steatotic liver)/hard (cirrhotic/fibrotic liver)
  ○ Spleen is enlarged or not
  If yes, measure size from costal margin along its long axis

Note its:
Extent: Up to mid-clavicular line/umbilicus/beyond umbilicus
- Surface: Margins; notch present or not
  ○ Consistency
  ○ Movement with respiration
- See if it is tender/nontender

Grading of splenomegaly by Hacketts method: from 0 to 5
- Grade 0: Unpalpable
- Grade 1: Palpable only on deep palpation
- Grade 2: Palpable until the midway point between costal margin and umbilicus
- Grade 3: Palpable beyond the midway point between costal margin and umbilicus
- Grade 4: Palpable beyond the umbilicus
- Grade 5: Reaching up to the pubic symphysis
  Any other palpable lump.

Make note of the direction of blood flow within dilated veins:
- Direction of blood flow in the peri-umbilical veins (Caput Medusae) in patients with portal hypertension is away from the umbilicus.

- Direction of blood flow in the flank veins:
  - Above downwards suggests superior vena cava (SVC) obstruction
  - Below upwards suggests inferior vena cava (IVC) obstruction
- Palpate groin hernia sites and examine genitals
- Look for tenderness in renal angles
- Examine back and spine for tenderness.

On percussion:
- Look for upper border of liver dullness (generally in the 5th intercostal space) in midclavicular line.
- Note the liver span (normal being 12–14 cm)
- *Length of splenic dullness*
- *Percussion in the Traube's space*: Left costal margin, left anterior axillary line and 6th rib form the boundaries of the Traube's space. Dull note in this space suggests splenomegaly.
- Note in the rest of the abdomen
- *Tests for free fluid*: Ascites present after hepatic decompensation of cirrhosis or transiently after bleed episode in NCPH (NCPF>>>EHPVO)

On auscultation:
- Look for bowel sounds, bruit hum and rub

Look for:
- *Kenawy sign*: Venous hum in the epigastric region due to flow in splenic vein
- *Cruveilhier–Baumgarten sign*: Venous hum in the umbilical region due to flow in recanalized umbilical vein (diagnostic of portal hypertension)
- *Proctoscopic evaluation*: To look for rectal varices

Rest systemic examination

Differential diagnosis include:
- NCPF
- EHPVO
- Chronic liver disease (CLD) (Child's A) **(Table 1)**

TABLE 1: Child's classification.[1]

Child–Turcotte–Pugh classification

	1 point	2 points	3 points
Encephalopathy	0	1–2	3–4
Ascites	None	Slight	Moderate
Bilirubin (mg/dL)	<2	2–3	>3
Albumin (g/dL)	>3.5	2.8–3.5	<2.8
PT prolonged (s)	1–4	5–6	>6
INR	<1.7	1.8–2.3	>2.3

- Child's A = 5–6 points
- Child's B = 7–9 points
- Child's C = 10–15 points

■ DEFINITIONS AND MANAGEMENT

- *Acute variceal bleed (AVB)*:
  - Active bleed from esophageal varices (EV)/gastric varices (GV) during upper gastrointestinal endoscopy (UGIE)
  - Presence of large EV/GV with blood in stomach
- *Clinically significant variceal bleed (VB)*:
  - HR >100
  - BP <100 or postural drop >20
  - >2 Packed red cells (PRCS) ≤ 24 hours from T0 (time of bleed)
- *Time frame for AVB*: T0 to 5 days
- *Failure to control AVB*:
  - Hematemesis/NG aspirate >100 mL fresh blood >2 hours of specific treatment
  - Hypovolemic shock
  - ≥ 3 g/dL drop in Hb ≤ 24 hours without PRCs
- *Variceal rebleeding*: Clinically significant rebleeding after 5 days
- *Clinically significant rebleeding*: Hematemesis/Melena needing—
  - Hospital admission
  - ≥ 3 g/dL drop in Hb
  - PRCs
  - Death within 6 weeks
- *Management of AVB*:
  - Secure airway, breathing, 2 wide bore angios, IV crystalloids, maintain mean arterial pressure (MAP) above 65, and mixed venous oxygen saturation (MVOS) above 70%.
  - Restrictive PRC transfusions, with target Hb 7–8
  - Transfuse platelets if <50 k, FFP if fibrinogen <1 g/dL
  - Insufficient evidence for tranexamic acid
  - Vasopressin + Glyceryl trinitrate: Reduction in failure to control bleed but not in mortality
  - Terlipressin: Improves survival as well.
    - Dose given as 2 mg 4–6 hourly as a continuous infusion for 5 days (as per Baveno V). May cause peripheral vasoconstriction with painful hands and feet.
  - Somatostatin/Octreotide can be used as well.
    - Octreotide: 100 mics bolus followed by 50 mics/hour infusion for 5 days.
- *Timing of UGIE*:
  - Immediately after stabilizing patient with severe AVB
  - For all AVB within 24 hours
- *For failure to achieve hemostasis, make use of*:
  - Sengstaken–Blakemore tube till next intervention: Endoscopic variceal ligation (EVL)/TIPS/Shunt/Devascularization surgery
  Deflate the balloon after 24 hours for 4 hours then inflate again for next 24 hours. Controls bleed in 90%. 50% rebleed after deflation. Serious complications like esophageal ulceration, aspiration pneumonia seen

in 20%. Esophageal balloon is rarely required and is never used on its own.
- Danis SX-ELLA fully covered SEMS: Can be left in place for 2 weeks, so oral intake/RT placement possible and it is good for post-endoscopic sclerotherapy (EST) ulcers, but is as expensive as transjugular intrahepatic portosystemic shunt (TIPS)]
- Hemostatic sprays (Ankaferd, Hemospray)

Now starting with the NCPH story:
Even when diagnosis of EHPVO is obvious after history, always say, you would like to give your diagnosis and differential diagnoses as follows:
- *Diagnosis*: Portal hypertension (PHTN) most likely non-cirrhotic in etiology, +/− bleeder, symptomatic splenomegaly, symptomatic hypersplenism, with symptomatic portal cavernoma cholangiopathy (PCC) (jaundice secondary to cholestasis, pain due to stones +/− cholangitis), delay in milestones/growth retardation/delay in sexual development/poor scholastic performance status endoscopic management.
- *Differential diagnoses (DDs)*: EHPVO, NCPF and chronic liver disease (Child's A). Remember that these are only your differentials. The final diagnosis will be known only on investigating further. Consider history as well, but generally, NCPF will have massive splenomegaly going beyond umbilicus (due to more proximal block), while EHPVO will have moderate splenomegaly.

Just remember that longstanding NCPF (up to 30%) can land up with CLD/cirrhosis, while longstanding EHPVO due to prolonged portal flow deprivation can have progressive deterioration of liver functions with reduced hepatic cell mass and synthetic function.

Also, NCPF and EHPVO both can land up with cirrhosis secondary to transfusion related HBV/HCV infection.

Why not Budd–Chiari syndrome (BCS) or right heart failure?
Because they present with painful hepatomegaly and ascites, followed by PHTN manifestations.

So without hepatomegaly and ascites, BCS and right heart failure (RHF) are unlikely.

Just remember that tender splenomegaly is seen in:
- Splenic infarct and abscess
- Typhoid
- Infectious endocarditis
- Infectious mononucleosis (EBV, CMV)

EHPVO Definition

As per the APASL consensus, EHPVO is defined as "a vascular disorder of liver, characterized by obstruction of the extrahepatic portal vein (PV) with or without involvement of intrahepatic PV radicles or splenic or superior mesenteric veins".[2]

APASL Criteria for NCPF/IPH[3]
- Presence of moderate to massive splenomegaly
- Evidence of portal hypertension, varices, and/or collaterals
- Patent splenoportal axis and hepatic veins on ultrasound
- Test results indicating normal or near—normal liver functions
- Normal or near—normal HVPG
- Liver histology—no evidence of cirrhosis or parenchymal injury

Other features:
- Absence of signs of chronic liver disease
- No decompensation after variceal bleed except occasional transient ascites
- Absence of serum markers of hepatitis B or C virus infection
- No known etiology of liver disease
- Imaging with ultrasound or other imaging techniques showing dilated and thickened portal vein with peripheral pruning and periportal hyperechoic areas

Portal Cavernoma Cholangiopathy (PCC) is Defined by the INASL[4]
As abnormalities in the extrahepatic biliary system including the cystic duct and gallbladder with or without abnormalities in the 1st and 2nd generation biliary ducts in a patient with portal cavernoma (PC). For the diagnosis to be established all of the following criteria would have to be fulfilled:
- Presence of a portal cavernoma
- Typical cholangiographic changes on ERC or magnetic resonance cholangiography
- Absence of other causes of these biliary changes like bile duct injury, primary sclerosing cholangitis, cholangiocarcinoma, etc.

■ INVESTIGATIONS TO DIAGNOSE

So sequence of investigations:
Blood tests, USG abdomen (to get diagnosis of type of NCPH and if CLD is present), followed by prothrombotic workup for EHPVO, viral markers, fibroscan and transjugular biopsy.

Then, UGIE for varices **(Tables 2 and 3)**. Finally CT/MR portovenogram (MR PV) (to plan surgery) and MRCP (to look for PCC).

The chief investigation to diagnose EHPVO and NCPF is USG abdomen with Doppler:

EHPVO: Presence of Portal Cavernoma with normal liver. IHBRD may be seen signifying PCC. If portal cavernoma seen, ask for prothrombotic workup which includes tests for—Protein C deficiency, protein S deficiency, anti-thrombin 3 deficiency, factor V Leiden mutation, prothrombin gene mutation, anticardiolipin antibody, lupus anticoagulant, antiphospholipid antibody, homocysteine levels, JAK-2 mutation.

CHAPTER 6: Non-cirrhotic Portal Hypertension

TABLE 2: Classification for grading of esophageal varices.[5]

Conn's classification	
Grade I	Visible only during one phase of respiration/performance of Valsalva manoeuvre
Grade II	Visible during both phases of respiration
Grade III	3–6 mm in diameter
Grade IV	>6 mm in diameter
Paquet's classification	
Grade I	Microcapillaries located in distal esophagus or esophagogastric junction
Grade II	One or two small varices located in the distal esophagus
Grade III	Medium-sized varices of any number
Grade IV	Large-sized varices in any part of esophagus
Westaby classification	
Grade 1	Varices appearing as slight protrusion above mucosa, which can be depressed with insufflations
Grade 2	Varices occupying <50% of the lumen
Grade 3	Varices occupying >50% of the lumen and which are very close to each other with confluent appearance

TABLE 3: Sarin classification of gastroesophageal varices.[5]

Gastroesophageal varices type 1	Continuation of esophageal varices into the lesser curvature (GOV1)
Gastroesophageal varices type 2	Esophageal and fundal varices are present in continuity with the greater curvature (GOV2)
Isolated gastric varices type 1	• Fundal varices are present in the cardia in the absence of esophageal varices (IGV1) • Indication for upfront surgery
Isolated gastric varices type 2	Fundal varices present in the stomach outside of cardio-fundal region or first part of duodenum (IGV2)

NCPF: Patent superior mesenteric vein (SMV), splenic vein (SV), portal vein (PV) and hepatic vein (HV), with thickened PV and peripheral pruning +/- altered liver echotexture.

Doppler is used to assess HV, flow and direction in portal system, flow in SMV/SV, size of SV and left renal vein (LRV). Even NCPF and cirrhosis can have PV thrombosis but in them PV is seen distinctly and there is no cavernoma, and also liver echotexture may be altered in these two.

The moment you see altered echotexture, think only of NCPF or cirrhosis. Long-standing EHPVO may lead to smaller left lobe (due to more commonly involved left portal vein secondary to thrombus extending from umbilical vein which drains into LPV), and deranged liver functions due to chronic portal flow deprivation (synthetic dysfunction showing low albumin and increased INR may be seen) and PCC (cholestasis/cholangitis picture). *But cirrhosis is not seen with EHPVO, unless* secondary to PCC or HBV/HCV (blood transfusion related). So just remember, if portal cavernoma is present, then diagnosis of EHPVO is confirmed, and if cirrhosis is also present due to these two causes, then final diagnosis will become EHPVO with secondary cirrhosis.

Now once this finding is seen, it has to be treated like CLD, whatever maybe the initial disease to start with. So now management changes as shunt may not be considered (it will lead to encephalopathy), and now to see status of liver, immediately ask for viral markers next, followed by fibroscan and transjugular liver biopsy. (If only fibrosis present, then shunt can be done. But if cirrhosis present, then shunt is contraindicated, and plan for splenectomy with devascularization with lifelong endoscopic management of symptomatic PCC if + or patient can be considered for transplant).

Then do UGIE—presence of varices/portal hypertensive gastropathy confirms the presence of portal hypertension.

Gastric varices cannot be banded as scope has to be retroflexed and it is not possible to band.

Post-endoscopic sclerotherapy there is periesophageal and perigastric fibrosis, and can lead to splenic vein (SV) thrombosis and calcification.

CT/MR PV with MRCP [to see HV, left PV status, portal cavernoma (PC) location and size, whether causing PCC, extension of thrombus into SMV/SV, collaterals, SV and LRV size] is a must before shunt.

■ SURGICAL INDICATIONS

Indications for surgery (PSRS whenever feasible/otherwise non-shunt surgery-devascularization to be done).

Absolute:
- Medically/endoscopically refractory variceal bleed and primary prophylaxis in EHPVO
- Secondary prophylaxis in NCPH
- Symptomatic splenomegaly, hypersplenism (recurrent bleeds or infections)
- Severe thrombocytopenia (platelet count <10,000/mm^3)
- Ectopic varices
- Symptomatic PCC

Relative:
- Poor health related QoL
- Large varices with poor access to healthcare or rare blood group
- Growth failure indication in children (Z-scores <2 despite nutritional rehabilitation)
- Delay in sexual development

TYPES OF SURGERIES FOR NCPH

Nonselective shunt: *PSRS (proximal splenorenal shunt)—splenectomy done and shunt performed (practically performed in an elective setting)*
- All the problems of NCPH like symptomatic splenomegaly, symptomatic hypersplenism, varices and ectopic varices, portal hypertensive gastro-enterocolopathy and symptomatic PCC are addressed and is the practical, durable and one time solution to solve the problems of NCPH. However, it cannot be done in absence of a shuntable vein (anatomical reason) and must not be done in presence of cirrhosis (propensity to lead to encephalopathy)

Selective shunt:
- Splenectomy not done and shunt performed
- Works similar to endoscopic variceal control, while rest of the problems of NCPH are not addressed (practically not performed).

DSRS: Warren shunt—distal splenorenal shunt.

Inokuchi shunt: Coronary-caval shunt.

Partial portacaval shunt: (Practically not performed).

Sarfeh shunt (8 mm interposition shunt)—maintains some prograde portal flow to liver.

Devascularization surgery: *Gastroesophageal variceal control + splenectomy (practically performed in an emergency setting for bleeding or in an elective setting in absence of a shuntable vein and in presence of cirrhosis)*

Original Sugiura–Futugava surgery:
- 2 stage
- Left thoracotomy sixth intercostal space (ICS)
- Lower 15 cm esophagus (inferior pulmonary vein – hiatus)
- Perforation veins ligated
- Esophageal transection
- Preserve collaterals
- After 4 weeks abdominal surgery
- Splenectomy
- Devascularization greater + lesser curvature (6–7 cm)
- Preserve left gastric vein
- Pyloroplasty, vagotomy

Modified Sugiura–Futugava surgery: One stage via abdominal approach

Mathur's modification of Sugiura:
- Abdominal surgery
- No splenectomy
- Lower 10 cm esophagus—disconnection of (perforators + collaterals)
- Esophageal transection

- Stomach—greater curvature (short gastric + left gastric epiploic)
- Lesser curvature (left gastric vein)
- Fundal varices—interlocking sutures
- Vagus preserved (if possible)
- Nissen fundoplication

Hassabs surgery:
- Abdominal
- Splenectomy
- Lower 10 cm esophagus (collaterals + perforators)
- Proximal half of stomach (short gastric + left gastric vein)
- No pyloroplasty/no esophagus transection
  (90% success—intramural connections not addressed—hence sclerotherapy)

Before surgery, get vaccination for splenectomy to prevent overwhelming post-splenectomy infection (OPSI) (Hib, pneumococcal in adults and additionally meningococcal in children).

For PSRS, 7 mm SV is enough, while LRV should be around 1 cm. Smaller RV can lead to eddy currents and thrombosis.

Post-shunt, antiplatelets (aspirin/clopidogrel) must be started if platelets go beyond 10 lakhs to prevent arterial thrombosis.

Consider long-term anticoagulation (6–12 months) with LMWH/Fondaparinux (oral Xa inhibitor) for cases with small RV/extensive thrombosis extending into SMV, etc., and lifelong anticoagulation for those with confirmed prothrombotic states.

Also if there was symptomatic PCC associated, then after shunt, do reimaging with USG and MR after 4–6 months to see if PCC has reversed. If not, patient needs second stage hepaticojejunostomy (HJ).

■ SPECIFIC POINTS FOR SURGERY FOR NCPH

1. Prophylactic shunt for EHPVO, but not for NCPF.
2. This is because, post-shunt surgery in NCPF, ~15% develop hepatopulmonary syndrome (HPS), nephropathy, myelopathy, and encephalopathy. Hence patients with NCPF should be carefully evaluated for the indication of surgery. Those with failed endotherapy and who are at high risk of re-bleeding [large varices, red color signs or isolated gastric varices (IGV)] should undergo a non-selective portosystemic shunt such as PSRS. However, those who have not had variceal bleeding or have low grade varices, but need surgery for symptomatic splenomegaly/hypersplenism should be managed with splenectomy and devascularization.
3. If minimal hepatic encephalopathy (MHE) (seen only with EHPVO in ~15%), HPS, portopulmonary hypertension (PPH) (seen less commonly with EHPVO) are present in EHPVO, all portosystemic shunts are contraindicated as they will worsen it all *except MESO-REX BYPASS* (porto-portal shunt), which is curative for it. If Rex shunt is not possible, then liver transplant is the only

treatment of choice. Also, for secondary biliary cirrhosis (SBC) in EHPVO, secondary to longstanding PCC, liver transplant is the treatment of choice.
4. If HPS, PPH (seen more commonly with NCPH) or cirrhosis happen in NCPF (seen in ~30% of longstanding disease), then liver transplant is the only treatment of choice. *(Graft can have portal blood inflow through a conduit to even a small segment of patent portal venous system or even to a cavernoma vessel).*

Remember that for EHPVO, the concern for delay in milestones/growth retardation/ delay in sexual development/poor scholastic performance is only in children. So by doing a Rex shunt, all of these can be prevented/reversed. Growth retardation in children after Rex shunt improves because spleen size reduces, so food intake increases, portal hypertensive enteropathy is taken care of, so food absorption improves, and growth hormone resistance goes down as portal flow to liver is restored, and thus levels of insulin like growth factor (IGF-1) and IGF-binding protein 3 rise again.

While for EHPVO in adults, it's too late to reverse these.
However, PSRS (nonselective shunt) in adults can still take care of symptomatic splenomegaly, symptomatic hypersplenism, varices and ectopic varices, portal hypertensive gastroenterocolopathy and symptomatic PCC. Also, substrate (food) utilization is improved after shunt surgery as huge spleen is removed, pain and early satiety improve and food consumption increases, and food absorption improves as portal hypertensive enteropathy is taken care of. But as mentioned above, if MHE, HPS, PPH are present, then the only option in EHPVO is a Rex shunt or transplant.

■ APPROACH TO THE MANAGEMENT OF MALIGNANCY IN THE PRESENCE OF NCPH

If suppose there is a gastric lesion along with NCPH, then get a biopsy and confirm it. If it is adenoCA, then get all imaging done starting from USG abdomen, CXR to CECT with CT portovenogram. Then completely stage the disease with PET CT and staging laparoscopy with peritoneal wash cytology.

Then MDT discussion.

Then do a PSRS, but if splenectomy was done previously, then splenic vein will be thrombosed, so then try to do a mesocaval shunt and after that in the time it takes to decompress the collaterals, plan NACT.

Then reassess with imaging, do staging laparoscopy again before surgery, and then proceed with D2 gastrectomy and complete the perioperative chemotherapy.

Now in this case, suppose a shunt is not possible, because of SMV-SV thrombosis, or unfavorable anatomy [and because a devascularization procedure does not decompress the portal cavernoma (PC) and hepatoduodenal ligament (HDL) and perioperative field collaterals, but in fact worsens it], then there are only two options available:
- Either resect in presence of collaterals (D1 can be done, as D2 will be dangerous in presence of collaterals along HDL and Splenic)

- Or plan for definitive chemotherapy/chemoradiotherapy and at the most do a devascularization procedure to at least take care of varices (but just remember that devascularization procedures will increase the risk of ectopic varices, portal hypertensive gastroenterocolopathy, and will worsen PCC)

■ REFERENCES

1. Pugh RN, Murray-Lyon IM, Dawson JL, Pietroni MC, Williams R. Transection of the oesophagus for bleeding oesophageal varices. Br J Surg. 1973;60(8):646-9.
2. Sarin SK, Sollano JD, Chawla YK, Amarapurkar D, Hamid S, Hashizume M, et al. Consensus on extra-hepatic portal vein obstruction. Liver Int. 2006;26(5):512-9.
3. Sarin SK, Kumar A, Chawla YK, Baijal SS, Dhiman RK, Jafri W, et al. Noncirrhotic portal fibrosis/idiopathic portal hypertension: APASL recommendations for diagnosis and treatment. Hepatol Int. 2007;1:398-413.
4. Dhiman RK, Saraswat VA, Valla DC, Chawla Y, Behera A, Varma V, et al. Portal cavernoma cholangiopathy: consensus statement of a working party of the Indian national association for study of the liver. J Clin Exp Hepatol. 2014;4:S2-14.
5. Abby Philips C, Sahney A. Oesophageal and gastric varices: historical aspects, classification and grading: everything in one place. Gastroenterol Rep (Oxf). 2016;4(3):186-95.

CHAPTER 7.1

Colorectal—Rectal Prolapse and Cancer

■ HISTORY

- *History of bleeding per rectum (PR)*:
  - Painful or painless: Hemorrhoids, rectal prolapse, polyposis, arteriovenous malformation (AVM) and colorectal cancer (CRC) cause painless PR bleed. Painful bleed suggests fissure in ano, thrombosed external hemorrhoids or inflammatory bowel disease.
  - History of passing fresh bright red or altered blood: Sigmoid/anorectal bleed appears fresh bright red whereas bleed from a more proximal site leads to passage of altered dark blood.
  - Blood separate from stools or mixed: Sigmoid/anorectal bleed appears separate from stools. Hemorrhoids cause bleeding which appears as drops of blood on the toilet bowl and occasionally may even be severe, whereas fissure in ano causes stripes of blood over stools. Whereas blood admixed with stools suggests bleed from a more proximal site.
  - Presence of blood clots: Suggests significant bleed
  - Frequency and volume: To gauge the blood loss
- *History of fatigue, shortness of breath, postural dizziness, syncope, need for blood transfusion*: To know the severity of bleed and presence of these features points to the presence of anemia
- *History to rule out UGI subacute intestinal obstruction secondary to Crohn's disease (CD)/intestinal TB (ITB)*: Ask for presence of abdominal pain, distension, ball rolling sensation, nausea, vomiting
- *History of alteration in bowel habits*: IBD presents with diarrhea. Carcinoma distal ascending colon/hepatic flexure/proximal transverse colon patients present with bleed per rectum (maroon colored stools) and they may land up with closed loop obstruction (due to distal obstruction by growth and proximally due to a functional IC valve) presenting with colicky abdominal pain, nausea, vomiting, constipation, obstipation due to which emergency management (colonoscopic stenting or proximal diversion with a stoma or hemicolectomy) is required, otherwise patient may land up with caecal perforation. Whereas Carcinoma rectum and left colon causes stricturing which obstructs the passage, leading to gradually increasing constipation.

- History of urgency, tenesmus (sensation of incomplete evacuation of bowels) and nocturnal defecation which are irritative rectal symptoms: Indicative of IBD or malignancy.
- History of spurious diarrhea: Colorectal cancer may lead to partial bowel obstruction, which results in the build-up of fluid and stool in the colon. This stagnant stool then liquifies, mixed with mucus proximal to the obstruction, to present as what is known as spurious diarrhea
- *History of perianal pain*: Indicative of fissure in ano/abscess
  - History of perianal discharge: Indicative of fistula in ano/ruptured abscess
  - History of mass per rectum: Indicative of either prolapsed internal hemorrhoids, external hemorrhoids, rectal prolapse or tumor. Ask whether it is soft (benign) or firm (neoplastic), prolapsing with straining (hemorrhoids/rectal prolapse) or not, reducible (hemorrhoids/rectal prolapse) or not and whether any history of incontinence
- *History of fecaluria is indicative of rectourinary/colo-urinary fistula.*
- *History of fever*: Will be seen in IBD, ITB
- *History of loss of weight (LOW), loss of appetite (LOA) are indicative of malignancy*
- *History of metastatic disease*:
  - Abdominal distension: Due to malignant ascites
  - Dry cough, hemoptysis: Due to pleural effusion and lung metastasis
  - Bony pain, non-traumatic fractures: Due to bony metastasis
  - Back pain: Due to vertebral metastasis
  - Unexplained sudden new onset headaches, blackouts, seizures: Due to brain metastasis

Treatment history: Whether CECT, colonoscopy, biopsy done and whether any surgery done in emergency for the present disease and whether chemotherapy and/or radiotherapy was given.

Family history (**Tables 1 and 2**):
- *Lynch syndrome*: Due to mismatch repair gene *(MLH1, MSH2, PMS2)* mutation
- *Familial adenomatous polyposis (FAP)*: Due to adenomatous polyposis coli *(APC)* gene mutation

TABLE 1: Amsterdam 2 criteria for HNPCC.[1]

At least three members of a family with hereditary nonpolyposis or associated (endometrial, small bowel, ureter or renal pelvis cancer) colorectal cancer and the following criteria must be met:	First degree of consanguinity in at least two of the affected members
	Clinical presentation in at least two consecutive generations
	Diagnosis of at least one case of colorectal cancer or associated cancers before age 50 years
	Discarded familial adenomatous polyposis
	Tumors verification through histopathology tests

CHAPTER 7.1: Colorectal—Rectal Prolapse and Cancer

TABLE 2: Revised Bethesda criteria for HNPCC.[2]

Tumors of individuals should be screened for microsatellite instability in the following situations:	CRC in a patient diagnosed before age 50 years
	Presence of synchronous, metachronous, or other HNPCC-associated tumors regardless of age
	CRC with high microsatellite instability (MSI-H) in a patient diagnosed before age 60 years
	CRC in one or more first-degree relatives with HNPCC or HNPCC-related tumor diagnosed before age 50 years
	CRC diagnosed in two or more of first- or second-degree relatives with HNPCC-related tumors regardless of age

(CRC: colorectal cancer; HNPCC: hereditary nonpolyposis colorectal cancer; MSI: microsatellite instability)

- *Peutz-Jeghers syndrome*: Due to *STK11* gene mutation
- *Juvenile polyposis syndrome*: Due to *SMAD4, BMPR1A* gene mutation
- *Cowden syndrome*: Due to *PTEN* gene mutation

Performance history: As per ECOG (Eastern Cooperative Oncology Group) classification to know if the patient will tolerate surgical stress or at least chemo/radiotherapy.

■ EXAMINATION PROFORMA

General Examination: Part A

- *Visual appearance*:
  - Young/middle aged/elderly
- *Gender*:
  - Male/female
- *Built*: Poor/average/good
- *Nourishment*: Poor/average/good
  - Measure height, weight, BMI
- *Clinical evaluation*:
  - Conscious/stuporous
  - Cooperative/uncooperative
  - Orientation to time, place and person: Present/absent
  - Hydration status: Hydrated/dehydrated
  - Lying comfortably bed/in discomfort/in pain
  - Whether patient prefers sitting or lying down position
  - Febrile/Afebrile
- *Vitals*: Pulse, BP, respiratory rate, mention performance status here as well

General Examination: Part B

Look for PICCLE, oral cavity [Peutz–Jeghers syndrome (PJS) macules], skin lesions (polyposis and IBD related).

PICCLE: Pallor, icterus, cyanosis, clubbing, generalized or localized lymphadenopathy, palpable cervical and left supraclavicular lymph node, pedal or dependent edema.

Skin lesions: Look for skin lesions like epidermoid cyst (filled with dead skin cells) which may be seen in Gardner syndrome, keratoacanthoma and sebaceous tumors which may be seen in Muir–Torre syndrome (variant of Lynch syndrome).

Examination of oral cavity: Oral hygiene, caries, any mucosal lesions. Look for hallmark of Peutz–Jeghers syndrome—pigmented macules on lips or oral mucosa. (In adults with PJS, skin macules may disappear but oral mucosal lesions persist).

Abdominal Examination

On inspection see if:
- Abdominal contour: Flat/distended/scaphoid
- Umbilicus: Central/displaced. Inverted/everted/flat
- All quadrants are moving equally with respiration or not
- Any visible lump/nodule
- *Look for*: Visible scar, sinus, engorged veins, pulsations, peristalsis or cough impulse
- Inspect the groin hernial sites and examine genitalia.
- Inspection of renal angles to look for fullness

On palpation: *See if*
- Abdomen is soft, nontender
- Liver is palpable or not (hepatomegaly may be present in case of liver metastasis)
- If palpable, measure its extent from costal margin in midclavicular line

See if:
- It is tender/nontender
- Consistency is soft/firm/hard
- Surface is smooth/nodular
- Borders are round/sharp, regular/irregular
- Margins
- Spleen is enlarged or not
  Carcinoma distal ascending colon/hepatic flexure/proximal transverse colon patients may land up with closed loop obstruction (due to distal obstruction by growth and proximally due to a functional IC valve) and a palpable firm cystic mass (distended colon)
- Palpate groin hernia sites and examine genitals
- Look for tenderness in renal angles
- Examine back and spine for tenderness.

On percussion:
- Look for upper border of liver dullness (generally in the 5th intercostal space) in midclavicular line
- Note the liver span (normal being 12–14 cm)

- Percussion note in the rest of the abdomen (generally tympanic)
- Tests for free fluid

On auscultation:
- Auscultate for bowel sounds. Hear for hyperperistaltic bowel sounds, if there is clinical suspicion of intestinal obstruction
- Auscultate for bruit, hum and rub

PER-RECTAL EXAMINATION PROFORMA

- Diaper or pad if being used
- Look for excoriation of perianal skin due to feces in a patient with incontinence or in a patient using diaper.
- Look for fissure, perianal abscess, sinus, external opening of fistula in ano, skin tag, external/internal hemorrhoids, growth or prolapse

Digital rectal examination:
- Mention tone and squeeze pressure as the first point. If the sphincter function is poor, then sphincter saving procedures should not be done.
- Assess distance of the growth from anal verge and anal ring.
- Assess the longitudinal and circumferential extent of the growth
- *Consistency*: Soft/firm/hard
- *Form*: Ulcerative/proliferative/ulcero-proliferative/polypoidal
- *Fixity*: Fixed or not
- *Note the staining on the gloved finger*: Normal stool/blood/mucus/pus.
- Proctoscopy to complete the examination.
  IBD → erythematous, inflamed, granular, friable mucosa with ulcers or erosion.
  Malignancy → all the above points and proximal and distal extent to be noted

Rest systemic examination

Before we embark on malignancy, let's review a completely benign entity before proceeding further.

CLINICAL CASE OF RECTAL PROLAPSE

Chief complaints: Something coming out of rectum
- *History of presenting illness (HOPI)*:
  - Since few months/years, during defecation and straining, mass was reducing by itself initially, but now requires digital manipulation to be reduced.
- *Ask for*:
  - Any pain/bleeding
  - Any abdominal pain, distention, ball rolling, nausea vomiting?
  - Any altered bowel habits (constipation/straining for hard stools/laxatives/diarrhea)
  - Ask for rectal irritative symptoms
  - Any incontinence to flatus/stools/feeling of wetness/soakage of undergarments.

- Any urinary symptoms (urgency, incontinence)
- If something coming out of vagina
- History of LOA, LOW and history indicative of metastatic disease to clinically orient yourself away from malignancy and toward a benign pathology
- *Then treatment history*: Any procedure performed for the present condition via abdominal/perineal route

Past history:
Comorbidities: Trauma, vaginal delivery, hysterectomy, pelvic surgery → etiology for rectal prolapse.

Personal: Married or not
- Children (live, type of delivery, prolonged labor → etiology for rectal prolapse)
- Family complete or not
- Sleep
- Appetite
- Diet
- Addiction
- Bowel bladder habits

Examination:
- *Detailed PR* examination as per proforma
- Then look for specific features:
  - Partial/full thickness prolapse (circumferential folds → rectal prolapse; longitudinal folds→hemorrhoids)
  - Appearance of mucosa (discoloration, erosions, ulcers, nodules, polyp, mass)
  - Reducible/not
  - Any other organ prolapse
  - Per vaginal (PV) exam
- DDs: Prolapse, mass, polyposis, hemorrhoids.

Management of Rectal Prolapse

Overview of investigations to be done: Colonoscopy [to rule out IBD, polyposis, mass], colonic transit study (to rule out colonic cause of constipation), baseline manometry [Rectoanal inhibitory reflex (RAIR) is continuously present in prolapse, so incontinence results], MR defecography (to rule out multicompartmental disease especially with history of vaginal delivery, pelvic trauma, previous pelvic surgery)

Investigations for rectal prolapse and constipation:
- Colonoscopy
- Colonic transit study (20 markers at 0, then at 12 and 24 hours. X-rays at 36 and 60 hours) to diagnose presence of slow transit constipation and fecal evacuation disorders
- Anorectal manometry with testing for rest, squeeze, push pressures and RAIR. (squeeze pressure >60 mm has better results after surgery)
- *Balloon expulsion test*: Normal ≤1 min

- MR defecography to look for degree of rectal prolapse and to look for associated anterior compartment defects like rectocele, enterocele, vaginal vault prolapse, cystocele during defecation. Also in evaluation of constipation, to diagnose anismus/puborectal dyssynergia (anorectal angle does not open >15°, paradoxical puborectalis contraction) and pelvic floor descent.

Surgical Indications

So remember that surgery is a must for colonic inertia (subtotal colectomy), anterior compartment defects (rectocele ≥2cm) and prolapse [ventral mesh rectopexy (VMR) is best]. Also for associated redundant sigmoid with prolapse, resection along with suture rectopexy must be done.

Whereas behavioral therapy, biofeedback, sacral nerve stimulation (SNS) should be used for the rest of the disorders.

If rectal prolapse presents with constipation/redundant sigmoid/diverticulosis, then patient needs sigmoid resection as well along with rectopexy.

If no prolapse, but constipation present due to slow colonic transit, then the treatment is subtotal colectomy.

If only prolapse with no pelvic descent, then VMR with a biodegradable mesh is the best procedure. Leeds study showed that biodegradable mesh had approximately 0% risk of mesh erosion versus 5% seen with prolene mesh. Also, posterior rectopexy can be done. However, with VMR as there is no posterior dissection, less constipation is seen, but if posterior rectopexy has been planned, then suture rectopexy is to be preferred over mesh as a Cochrane meta-analysis has shown equal recurrence between the two.

PROSPER trial: Equal recurrence rates between perineal and abdominal rectopexy. However, if there is prolapse with perineal descent/multicompartmental disease/recurrence after perineal surgery:
- *VMR is treatment of choice*: As it includes preservation of nerve plexi + closure of peritoneum over mesh + reinforcement of rectovaginal septum + correction of enterocele + correction of genital prolapse with sacrocolpopexy.
- *Postoperative advice*: High fiber diet, stool softener, laxatives, pelvic floor exercises. In 70% of patients, within 1–2 years, symptoms settle.

■ DDs FOR BLEED PR MIXED WITH STOOLS

- IBD [Ulcerative colitis (UC) >Crohn's]
- IBD with malignancy, *only* if there is a chronic history of 8–10 years of pan/left sided colitis with LOA and LOW
- Polyposis/Lynch syndromes
- Polyposis/Lynch with malignancy if age >35
- TB always consider in India. Also consider internal hemorrhoids in painless bleed in young
- Primary colorectal malignancy (lower down in young, but higher up in elderly)
  Remember that, Crohn's and TB will always present with features of subacute intestinal obstruction (SAIO): Colicky abdomen pain, distention, ball rolling,

nausea, vomiting, and also LOW, whereas, ulcerative colitis (UC) will generally always have bloody diarrhea.

Ulcers and benign strictures are more often seen in Crohn's, whereas stricture in UC is most often cancer.

■ COLORECTAL CANCER (CRC)

Ask for investigations in the following order:
- First, any previous Lower GI endoscopy (LGIE)/CECT report.
- Then two sets of investigations, first to assist in diagnosis, staging of disease, and other to complete the workup.

Diagnosis and Staging

In general, for diagnosis, if any luminal pathology is suspected, better do upper GI (UGI)/lower GI (LGI) scopy first with biopsy, followed by USG abdomen, CXR and then CECT (helps to get diagnosis fast and also helps where to look for lesion in CECT) +/−MR.

If growth is not obstructing, give full bowel preparation and then first do LGIE and biopsy. On the preoperative biopsy, do IHC for mismatch repair (MMR) or PCR for microsatellite instability (MSI) [So if MLH1 mutated or MSI positive, test for BRAF V600E mutation, because if that is present, then it is sporadic cancer due to hypermethylation of MLH1 whereas, if it is BRAF wild, then do germline testing for other MMR genes (MSH2, 6, PMS2 and EPCAM) and if present, then it is Lynch. Also microsatellite high (MSI-H) tumors do not respond to 5-FU, so Oxaliplatin must be added, though they have better prognosis due to high number of tumor infiltrating lymphocytes] and APC germline testing to know diagnosis (sporadic/Lynch/FAP), for screening [If Lynch+: screening colonoscopy at 20 years, endometrial biopsy and transvaginal ultrasound (TVUS) of ovaries at 25 years, urine cytology at 30 years, UGIE for gastric cancer at 30 years. If FAP+: screening colon at 10 years, prophylactic Colectomy, UGIE at 20 years. Look for congenital hypertrophic retinal pigment epithelium (CHRPE), thyroid, pancreas, CNS], and to select proper surgical plan so for Lynch: subtotal Colectomy with total abdominal hysterectomy with bilateral salpingo-oophorectomy (TAH BSO) and for Polyposis: Total proctocolectomy (TPC) and finally for genetic counseling. Check for KRAS/BRAF mutations, as after NAC/CRT, it may not be possible to get this information which is useful in a metastatic setting

Then blood tests with CEA:
- It is tumor marker used in the evaluation of colorectal cancer.
- *Normal level*: < 4 ng/mL
- Levels are raised in smokers
- *Role*:
  - Support diagnosis
  - Staging
  - Prognostication

- ○ Response assessment: Postneoadjuvant therapy, postsurgery, post-adjuvant
- ○ Surveillance
- Followed by USG abdomen pelvis, CXR to rule out unresectable metastases and then CECT with IV, oral and rectal contrast.
- *For rectal cancer*: CECT chest abdomen and MRI pelvis.
- *MRI pelvis protocol for rectal CA*:
  - ○ 1.5/3 Tesla, phased array coil
  - ○ No rectal contrast to be given (normal wall thickness <3 mm),
  - ○ High-resolution T2 images without fat suppression (to see mesorectal fat) taken in supine, three views: Sagittal, oblique coronal and oblique axial), with wide field of view upto aortic bifurcation.
  - ○ +/- T1 pre- and postgadolinium [~24% downstage of T stage, better diagnosis of extramural vascular invasion (EMVI)]
  - ○ +/- Diffusion weighted imaging (DWI)
  - ○ +/- Buscopan/Glucagon to reduce motion artefacts

The sagittal sections are reviewed to note the length of tumor, relation of tumor to the peritoneal reflection, involvement of anterior and posterior organs and to prepare oblique axial sections. In coronal sections relation of the tumor to levator ani, sphincters and pelvic side walls is noted. In oblique axial views the exact T and N stage is noted. T3 tumors are then further subclassified based on the depth of mesorectal invasion into T3a (<1 mm), T3b (1-5 mm), T3c (5-15 mm) and T3d (> 15 mm). Circumferential resection margin (CRM) is noted

MRI pelvis best for: T, N, EMVI, CRM [is considered to be involved if T/N/EMVI ≤ 1 mm of mesorectal fascia (MRF)], involvement of intersphincteric space/levators/puborectalis/external anal sphincter (EAS) and pelvic sidewall lymph nodes (PSWLN) (15% vs. 8% in low vs. high rectal cancer).

EUS: Endoscopic ultrasound—useful modality for T and N staging only if endoscopic mucosal resection (EMR)/endoscopic submucosal dissection (ESD) is being planned for early T1 disease.

Special tests: If endoluminal disease (ITB/IBD) suspected, CT/MR colonography is the best: Full bowel preparation given the day prior and positive contrast given orally without IV contrast and CO_2 per rectally (PR) for distention

If growth is obstructing then:
- No bowel preparation for colonoscopy (only enema)
- No oral contrast for CECT (only IV)
  Rest same

Now if preoperative CECT shows liver metastases, then get a FDG PET CT to rule out unresectable extrahepatic and extrapulmonary disease. *DW-MRI* will be more sensitive and specific for lesions <1 cm.

Other indications for FDG PET CT:
- Before exenteration surgery
- Also: High CEA, EMVI + on MRI (markers of high risk of metastases) and IV contrast allergy

Staging laparoscopy: May be done to look for peritoneal metastasis/occult liver metastasis which may be missed on preoperative imaging, and if positive, calculate peritoneal carcinomatosis index score (PCI). CRS + HIPEC can be done for PCI ≤15.

Management Principles of Colon Cancer as per ASCRS 4th Edition

Surgical resection of the primary tumor remains the cornerstone of treatment for stage I–III colon cancer and plays a role in treating surgically resectable stage IV disease.

At least a 5-cm margin should be obtained both proximally and distally, and the feeding vessel should be taken at its origin.

Lymphadenectomy is considered adequate when feeding vessels are taken at their origin and at least 12 lymph nodes have been harvested and examined histologically.

The aim of the mesocolic resection is to remove the tumor, its associated lymphovascular supply, including central vascular ligation (CVL), and mesocolon in an intact envelope of visceral peritoneum.

By performing a central ligation of the vessels, complete mesocolic excision (CME) also obtains central and apical lymph nodes and thus captures "skip lesions," which can occur in 5% of cases on average.[3-5] Completion of CME with an intact peritoneal lining has been demonstrated to improve survival by 15%.[6]

Adhesions from the tumor to other structures are malignant in about 40% of cases. If there is an uncertainty if there is direct invasion or rather merely abutment, proceeding with en bloc resection is favored. Without en bloc resection, patients are at higher risk of recurrence and decreased survival.[7]

Data from the FOxTROT Collaborative Group showed significant tumor downstaging, less apical node involvement, and fewer positive margins, thus, favoring preoperative treatment in patients with locally advanced, resectable colon cancer.[8] National Comprehensive Cancer Network (NCCN) also recommends consideration of neoadjuvant therapy in clinical T4b colon cancer, as this may improve survival.[9] Neoadjuvant chemoradiotherapy (NACRT) can be considered for sigmoid tumors invading the bladder or other pelvic organs, provided that the radiation dose to surrounding small bowel can be limited. NACRT has also been administered to select patients with more proximal colon tumors invading other vital structures such as duodenum and pancreas, although data are limited to case reports and small series.

Description of Surgical Procedures for CRC as per ASCRS

Surgery for Cecum and Ascending Colon Cancer

Right hemicolectomy (Ileocolic + right colic + right branch of middle colic).

Surgery for Hepatic Flexure Colon Cancer

Extended right hemicolectomy (Ileocolic + right colic + middle colic).

Surgery for Transverse Colon Cancer
Extended right or extended left hemicolectomy (left colic + middle colic) or transverse colectomy.

Surgery for Splenic Flexure Colon Cancer
Segmental left hemicolectomy (left branch of middle colic + left colic).

Surgery for Descending Colon Cancer
Formal left hemicolectomy (left branch of middle colic + IMA at root).

Surgery for Sigmoid Colon Cancer
- *Sigmoid colectomy/anterior resection*: (Superior hemorrhoidal artery giving sigmoidal arteries ligated, left colic arising from IMA preserved).
- Similar oncologic results as a formal left hemicolectomy done for sigmoid cancer.
- Rectum transected above level of peritoneal reflection

Role of Chemotherapy
All patients with resected stage III, and most with high-risk stage II, colon cancer should be considered for adjuvant chemotherapy for 3-6 months.

IDEA trial: 13,000 stage 3 randomized to 3 or 6 months of adjuvant CAPOX or FOLFOX. For low-risk stage 3 (T1–3/N1), 3 months CAPOX is non-inferior to 6. But 3 months FOLFOX is inferior to 6. Whereas for high-risk stage 3 (T4/N2), 3 months of both CAPOX or FOLFOX are inferior to 6. Based on this, NCCN recommends 3 months CAPOX OR 6 months FOLFOX for low-risk stage 3, but 6 months CAPOX OR FOLFOX for high-risk stage 3.

NSABP, MOSAIC, ASCO: For high-risk stage 2 (T4, obstructed, perforated, <12 LN harvested, poorly differentiated, close margins, tumor budding/LVI/PNI+):
- Capecitabine or 5-FU/Leucovorin adjuvant chemo must be given. Oxaliplatin must be added if tumor is MMR deficient as it would not be respond to 5-FU alone.

Management Principles of Rectal Cancer
NCCN 2020 Guidelines
Total 6 months of perioperative therapy either total neoadjuvant therapy (TNT) or the usual trimodal regimen of NACRT-surgery-chemo may be given.

For stage II/III mid and low rectal cancer, short-course radiotherapy (SCRT) (not for T4 if given solo, i.e., if not part of TNT) or long-course chemoradiotherapy (LC-CRT) followed by surgery, and systemic chemo given either before (becomes TNT) or after surgery (usual trimodal regimen).

They recommend adjuvant chemo for clinical stage II/III rectal cancer who received neoadjuvant radiation, regardless of final histology.

Now for deciding SCRT versus LC-CRT as part of USUAL TRIMODAL REGIMEN,
So LC-CRT preferred for T4/threatened or positive CRM, as it sterilizes, downstages and increases chance of organ preservation, whereas SCRT only sterilizes.

However, SCRT when used as part of TNT, is a valid treatment option for all advanced tumors (T3/4, N+, EMVI+, CRM+, pelvic side wall N+) and has been used in all consolidation versus standard trials.

Consolidation Chemo Landmark Trial

Angelita Habr-Gama's refined TNT protocol for T3/4 and/or N+ rectal cancers: Infusional 5-FU and Leucovorin 3 cycles-based 45 Grays RT over 5 weeks with 9 Grays boost followed by 3 cycles of infusional 5FU/Leucovorin, followed by tumor assessment after 8 weeks, with latest report showing clinical complete response (cCR) of 68%, with 5 years disease-free survival (DFS) of 60%.

TNT advantages: Higher compliance and systemic chemo completion, higher cCR—enabling watch and wait (WW) for organ preservation, higher pathological complete response (pCR)—almost double and pCR in consolidation >>induction, lower margin positivity rates, lower loco regional recurrence rates, lower distant metastases rate, and thus better DFS.

TNT is generally followed by surgery:
- Now if with advanced tumors/high-risk features (indication for preoperative chemoRT), cCR is seen, then there is an option of WW, which becomes accidental WW.
- But if the patient desires organ preservation for mid/low rectal tumors, then even if there is no indication for preoperative chemoRT (i.e., early tumors/no high-risk features), intentional WW with a view to organ preservation can be done using TNT.

Surgery for Rectal Cancer

Local excision alone [transanal endoscopic microsurgery (TEM) or Transanal minimally invasive surgery (TAMIS)] can be offered to patients with early T1 rectal cancers in the absence of adverse histopathologic features, such as poor differentiation, lymphovascular invasion (LVI), tumor budding, or close margins. Patients with low-risk T2 tumor should be considered for local excision only in the context of palliative intent or enrolment in a clinical trial.

NCCN guidelines clearly recommend local excision as the treatment of choice for: (1) mobile/nonfixed rectal tumors, (2) less than 3 cm in size, (3) occuping less than one-third of the circumference of the bowel, (4) not extending beyond the submucosa (T1) which are (5) well to moderately differentiated and (6) with low-risk histopathological features.

On the other hand, local excision should be avoided in cases of lymphovascular invasion, perineural invasion and mucinous components which are considered as high-risk characteristics, with high lymphnode metastatic potential.

According to the NCCN guidelines, the standard treatment for T2N0M0 rectal adenocarcinoma is Total Mesorectal Excision (TME) without adjuvant therapy.

The standard surgery for rectal cancer, however is proctectomy using the philosophy of TME.
- TME: The complete excision of the contents of the mesorectal envelope at risk for mesorectal metastases is the driving principle of proctectomy. It is the sharp dissection along these planes and the intact removal of the mesorectum and the contents therein that minimizes the risk of local recurrence.
- Rectal cancer with less than a 1 mm circumferential resection margin (<1 mm considered a positive resection margin) has a greater than 50% local recurrence rate.

Low anterior resection: Rectum transected below level of peritoneal reflection.

Ultra low anterior resection: Rectum transected at level of levator ani with anastomosis at level of dentate line.

Inter-sphincteric resection (ISR): Rectum transected below level of levator ani with dissection in the inter-sphincteric plane.

It is a procedure aimed at tumors of the lower rectum that can usually be assessed digitally as they are within 4–8 cm from the anus. Indications include carcinomas, villous adenomas, carcinoids and hemangiomas. Contraindications are undifferentiated cancers, T4 tumors and those that have invaded the sphincter apparatus.[10] Relative contraindications are those with poor sphincter function. Intersphincteric resection is a two-stage procedure comprising a perineal dissection in the intersphincteric plane and an abdominal component with TME to meet the dissection from below.[11] The internal sphincter is removed with the specimen leaving the external sphincter to aid in postoperative continence function. The final stage is a hand-sewn coloanal anastomosis. The abdominal component can be performed open, laparoscopically or robotic-assisted.

Transanal total mesorectal excision (taTME) helps in the most troublesome part of a minimally invasive proctectomy, i.e., the final 3–6 cm of distal rectal dissection and distal rectal transection. It is described as a two-team simultaneous approach. One team works laparoscopically from the abdomen to mobilize the colon and splenic fexure, ligate the IMA and IMV, and mobilize the upper half of the rectum. The other team works via a transanal approach by first starting with a circumferential full-thickness transection beginning in the intersphincteric plane and proceeding in a cephalad direction up to the top of the anorectal ring

Abdomino-perineal resection (APR): For low rectal cancers not meeting criteria for ISR—T4, PDAC, poor sphincter function

Classical APR: Waisting of specimen occurs as it keeps levators in place

Extra-levator abdomino-perineal excision (ELAPE): Specimen includes levators as well

Done to reduce incidence of CRM positivity and intraoperative bowel perforation, however mixed results seen in comparison with classical APR. Increased morbidity due to wound complications—leaves a huge perineal defect which cannot be closed.

Adjuvant therapy when NAC/CRT not given (tumor mis-staged by MRI ~25–30%), NCCN 2020 guidelines:
- *Total 6 months of therapy.*
- For low-risk stage II (pT3, negative CRM), adjuvant chemoRT followed by capecitabine OR 5-FU/leucovorin is preferred, but observation alone is also an option.
- For high-risk stage II (pT4, positive CRM, positive margins) or any stage III, adjuvant chemoRT followed by CAPOX or FOLFOX is preferred.

However, many argue that benefit of postoperative RT may be minimal if negative CRM and margins are achieved as compared to it's toxicity, and that current chemo regimens are highly effective. Thus, another reasonable strategy is to treat N+ but negative CRM and margins, with postoperative chemo only.

So now in case of M1 disease, if lung and liver metastases are resectable and there's no disease spread elsewhere, go for definitive treatment.

■ COLORECTAL LIVER METASTASES (CRLM)[12]

The EGOSLIM consensus group suggested a terminology of synchronous liver metastases (detected at or before diagnosis of the primary tumor), early metachronous metastases (detected within 12 months after diagnosis or surgery of the primary) and late metachronous metastases (detected > 12 months of diagnosis or surgery of primary).

Metachronous CRLM Management[13]

For CRLM, if Fong score ≤ 2 then go for upfront resection. But if ≥ 3 then NACT recommended. Otherwise generally, NACT is not recommended for upfront resectable CRLM as it increases hepatic toxicity in form of chemotherapy associated steatohepatitis (CASH) and sinusoidal obstruction syndrome (SOS), but doesn't add to better progression free survival (PFS) and overall survival (OS). However, NACT must be given for unequivocally unresectable CRLM and also to downstage disease to make it resectable, but < 6 cycles of CAPOX/FOLFOX/FOLFIRI must be given, as more increase toxicity. FOLFOXIRI has 25% better OS, at cost of increased toxicity. Also, targeted therapy can be added for better downstaging rates.

For CRLM with left sided primary: EGFR blockade (cetuximab, panitumumab) and even EGFR tyrosine kinase inhibitors (TKI): Erlotinib, gefitinib increase OS if RAS and BRAF wild type and are thus used with chemo, whereas they can reduce OS if used for right sided ones and thus are prohibited in them.

Also, for CRLM with left sided primary, if RAS, BRAF are mutated (downstream of EGFR), then anti-EGFR no benefit, but foll. can be used to increase OS:
1. If RAS mutated, add selumetinib
2. If BRAF mutated, add vemuRAFinib

Remember that BRAF mutations (R>L) in CRLM confer poor prognosis as they lead to multicentric recurrence after resection of CRLM signifying aggressive biology.

For CRLM with right sided primary: Anti-angiogenics like bevacizumab increase OS and are used with chemo.

OSLO COMET trial for laparoscopic versus open resection of CRLM:[14] So lap resection is non-inferior in terms of operative mortality, margin negativity and OS for both minor and major resections. Also, reduced postoperative pain, need for blood transfusion and length of stay.

Trials of orthotopic liver transplant (OLT) for unresectable liver-only CRLM:
- SECA 1 study: Poor OS as they included all tumors, so 4 poor prognostic factors: Liver tumor size >5.5 cm, CEA >80, interval from primary surgery to transplant <2 years, with progression of metastases on NACT.
- So SECA 2 trial done with these selective inclusion criteria, having better results, with 5 years OS of 83%.
- Ongoing SECA 3 and TRANSMET trials compare OLT versus systemic chemo for unresectable CRLM.

Synchronous CRLM Management[13]

Simultaneous liver and colon surgery: Consistent message from available studies is that simultaneous colon and liver resection (<3 segments) can be done safely in selected patients.

Indications for liver first surgery:
- Following downsizing of initially unresectable liver metastases with an asymptomatic primary tumor in situ, when it is deemed that there is a limited time window for successful liver resection
- In the situation of synchronous operable primary and colorectal liver metastases where the colorectal liver metastases may become inoperable during time taken to complete a primary first treatment plan
- In the specific instance of synchronous rectal cancer and liver metastases where the significant time interval between irradiation of the primary tumor and its resection (3-month window after long-course irradiation) gives an opportunity for metastases to be resected sooner than would be achieved if waiting till after resection of the primary.

Different scenarios for CRLM management:
- *Asymptomatic primary and unequivocally unresectable liver metastases.* In this scenario there is consensus to treat with upfront chemotherapy combined with EGFR blockade/anti-angiogenic agents, guided by principles as described above, with the intention of achieving maximal response, survival, and in some cases conversion to a resectable scenario for the liver metastases. For those patients who are converted to operability, liver first surgery may be considered over colon first.

- *Symptomatic primary and unequivocally unresectable liver metastases.* In this instance, the objective is to deal with symptoms from the primary, and then offer optimal systemic chemo. Bleeding may respond to systemic chemo and may be managed by blood transfusion. Obstruction may require proximal stoma/stenting/resection of the primary tumor. Perforation will usually mandate primary resection. Once primary's symptoms have been addressed, do as above.
- *Asymptomatic primary and resectable liver metastases.*

  Although the EGOSLIM consensus group recommended systemic chemo first for this scenario, there was no unanimity and evidence was lacking.[15]

  The only randomized evidence in this area comes from the EORTC 40983 trial[16] comparing surgery alone to FOLFOX-surgery FOLFOX, which showed an improved DFS in the perioperative chemo group, though no OS advantage in the early or long term.[17]

  However, it is difficult to state whether any survival advantage was associated with NACT, adjuvant, or both. Arguing against the value of NACT, Adam et al., showed no benefit associated with NACT prior to resection of solitary metachronous liver metastases.[15]

  Although providing some evidence, both Adam's study and the EORTC trial are not directly applicable to the scenario of synchronous liver metastases, as almost two-thirds of the liver metastases in the EORTC trial were metachronous, and Adam's study relates exclusively to metachronous liver metastases. In a retrospective report Bonney et al.[18] studied 1,301 patients with synchronous liver metastases, and compared those who received NACT prior to liver resection to those who underwent liver surgery without NACT. They found that for patients with solitary CRLM, neither NACT nor adjuvant chemo was associated with a survival advantage. In contrast, for patients with multiple liver metastases, although NACT conferred no benefit, adjuvant chemo was found to be associated with a survival advantage. In summary, current evidence certainly does not justify NACT in all cases of synchronous resectable liver metastases.
- *Symptomatic primary and resectable liver metastases.* In this scenario, priority is given to dealing with symptoms from the primary. Thereafter the next most appropriate treatment depends on the results of restaging. If restaging shows progression with now unresectable liver metastases, clearly chemo is indicated. If restaging suggests disease progression in the liver though still resectable, then a period of systemic chemo may be most appropriate to re-establish disease stability prior to reassessing with a view to liver resection. If restaging suggests stable and resectable metastases, then the scenario becomes similar in principle to the situation of "resectable primary and resectable liver metastases"

■ CRC WITH POLYPS (LYNCH OR FAP)

Make all efforts to first diagnose if it's Lynch or FAP, so if cost is not an issue, do preoperative IHC/PCR for MMR/MSI, followed by germline testing for *MMR/APC* genes.

If on preoperative imaging, cancer is locally advanced, plan for NAC/CRT, restage and then plan for definitive surgery and adjuvant chemo OR TNT for rectal cancer.

Before treatment, advise for sperm/ovum banking as RT will lead to sterilization.

Also, inform and take proper consent regarding postoperative possible urinary, sexual dysfunction, low anterior resection syndrome (LARS) and need for permanent stoma.

Then counsel the patient that he/she requires TPC with Ileal pouch anal anastomosis (IPAA) TWO-stage for familial adenomatous polyposis (FAP) OR subtotal colectomy with TAH and BSO if Lynch+, as postoperative biopsy will need to be analyzed to see if disease is locally advanced or not. Because if it is, then patient definitely needs adjuvant chemo (unless TNT received for rectal cancer) and then if one stage was done and if anastomosis leaks, then adjuvant therapy will get delayed, and every 4 week delay decreases OS by 14% (ASCRS 4th edition).

In a case of FAP planned for TPC with IPAA, first clear the rectum and anal transition zone (ATZ) of all polyps endoscopically, review their biopsy, and then proceed with IPAA. Because if any rectal polyp ≤1 cm from anorectal ring is positive for cancer, then ISR or even APR with a permanent stoma may need to be done.

Also if it's a young female, with high rectal polyp load, first do TPC with stoma, and do IPAA at a later date after she completes her family.

Also if rectal polyps are less than 20 and can be cleared endoscopically, do that, review the HPE of the polyps and then do TPC with IRA, start her on sulindac/celecoxib, and put rectum on surveillance every 6 monthly, as we need to preserve her urinary and sexual functions, fecundity and continence. After family completion, plan for completion proctectomy with IPAA.

FAP/IBD surgery: Before surgery in young, counsel for sperm/ovum banking, then post-TPC: Urinary, sexual dysfunction (reduced fecundity), incontinence, also post-IPAA: pouch related problems, pouchitis and also need for permanent stoma.

For FAP and Familial Juvenile Polyposis Syndrome (FJPS), TPC is compulsory, however IPAA or permanent stoma is patients choice. If sphincters are normal, then IPAA, and if not, then obviously end stoma.

Also in a young patient, we can still opt for Ileorectal anastomosis (IRA) (after endoscopic clearance of all rectal and ATZ polyps, and only after reviewing their histology), start sulindac/celecoxib for regression of rectal load and 6 monthly surveillance of rectum and then do completion proctectomy and IPAA once family is complete, however, TPC is the recommended procedure of choice in all patients of FAP and Juvenile Polyposis.

Also, for ulcerative colitis (UC), TPC is standard of care in elective and subtotal colectomy in emergency. However, for young patients of UC, subtotal colectomy can be done even in elective and rectum can be put on surveillance and then proctectomy and IPAA can be done after family is complete.

Three-stage TPC with IPAA: High steroid dose/toxic megacolon previously operated in emergency/young patient wants family first, pouch later.

Remember that as per textbook:
- *For all cases of polyposis, clear rectum and ATZ of polyps, review their histology and only then can proceed for restorative total proctocolectomy (TPC).*

    If it's a case of FAP or FJPS, then TPC (+/– IPAA) has to be done.

    For attenuated FAP (AFAP) with rectal sparing (or if <20 rectal adenomas are there) and also MUTYH polyposis, IRA can be done, sulindac/celecoxib is started, with rectum put on surveillance 6 monthly. At a later date, completion proctectomy with IPAA can be done for them.

    Even after IPAA, colonoscopic surveillance must be done as polyps may develop in anal transition zone (ATZ)/pouch, and ATZ carcinoma is known to occur even after 15 years, and hand sewn anastomosis after mucosectomy doesn't completely eliminate risk of subsequent polyposis and CA.
- Also for UC, TPC must be done in elective, and subtotal colectomy in emergency with completion proctectomy later. But for young patients of UC, subtotal colectomy can be done even in elective and rectum can be put on surveillance and then proctectomy and pouch can be done after family is complete.

However if there's a CRC associated with UC and also if diagnosis of UC is not sure, that is, if it can be UC or Crohn's, then pouch must be deferred till final histopathological examination report (HPE) is available. Because final HPE will tell two things: What kind of IBD it is and if adjuvant chemo/CRT is required or not. Because if it's Crohn's, then pouch is anyway contraindicated. However if it is UC, then after completing chemo/CRT, plan for IPAA if sphincters are normal or just end ileostomy (if continence is impaired before surgery or if patient desires it to avoid pouch related problems).

Surveillance of Operated CRC

Digital rectal examination (DRE), colonoscopy, *MRI (for local), CEA (marker of residual disease/recurrence), CECT/PET (for systemic metastases).*

■ LOW ANTERIOR RESECTION SYNDROME (LARS)

Risk factors: Preoperative radiotherapy (RT), complete total mesorectal excision (TME), intersphincteric resection (ISR), internal anal sphincter (IAS) damage, loss of RAIR, loss of rectal reservoir, denervation of neorectum, low height of anastomosis from anal verge, leak/sepsis.

Diagnosis: Wexner score, fecal incontinence severity index (FISI), LARS score (incontinence for flatus/liquids/solids, pad usage, QOL).

Management: Bulking, loperamide, 5-HT3 blocker (ramosetron), pelvic floor training, retrograde irrigation, biofeedback, balloon training, sacral nerve stimulation (SNS), tibial nerve stimulation, and stoma as last resort.

REFERENCES

1. Vasen HF, Watson P, Mecklin JP, Lynch HT. New clinical criteria for hereditary nonpolyposis colorectal cancer (HNPCC, Lynch syndrome) proposed by the International Collaborative group on HNPCC. Gastroenterology. 1999;116(6):1453-6.
2. Shia J, Holck S, DePetris G, Greenson JK, Klimstra DS. Lynch syndrome-associated neoplasms: a discussion on histopathology and immunohistochemistry. Fam Cancer. 2013;12:241-60.
3. Liang JT, Huang KC, Lai HS, Lee PH, Sun CT. Oncologic results of laparoscopic D3 lymphadenectomy for male sigmoid and upper rectal cancer with clinically positive lymph nodes. Ann Surg Oncol. 2007;14:1980-90.
4. Liang JT, Lai HS, Huang J, Sun CT. Long-term oncologic results of laparoscopic D3 lymphadenectomy with complete mesocolic excision for right-sided colon cancer with clinically positive lymph nodes. Surg Endosc. 2015;29:2394-401.
5. Siani LM, Lucchi A, Berti P, Garulli G. Laparoscopic complete mesocolic excision with central vascular ligation in 600 right total mesocolectomies: Safety, prognostic factors and oncologic outcome. Am J Surg. 2017;214(2):222-7.
6. West NP, Kobayashi H, Takahashi K, Perrakis A, Weber K, Hohenberger W, et al. Understanding optimal colonic cancer surgery: comparison of Japanese D3 resection and European complete mesocolic excision with central vascular ligation. J Clin Oncol. 2012;30(15):1763-9.
7. Lopez MJ, Monafo WW. Role of extended resection in the initial treatment of locally advanced colorectal carcinoma. Surgery. 1993;113(4):365-72.
8. Zhou Z, Nimeiri HS, Benson III AB. Preoperative chemotherapy for locally advanced resectable colon cancer-a new treatment paradigm in colon cancer?. Ann Transl Med. 2013;1(2):11.
9. Dehal A, Graff-Baker AN, Vuong B, Fischer T, Klempner SJ, Chang SC, et al. Neoadjuvant chemotherapy improves survival in patients with clinical T4b colon cancer. J Gastrointest Surg. 2018;22(2):242-9.
10. Martin ST, Heneghan HM, Winter DC. Systematic review of outcomes after intersphincteric resection for low rectal cancer. Br J Surg. 2012;99(5):603-12.
11. Heald RJ, Husband EM, Ryall RD. The mesorectum in rectal cancer surgery—the clue to pelvic recurrence?. Br J Surg. 1982;69(10):613-6.
12. Adam R, de Gramont A, Figueras J, Kokudo N, Kunstlinger F, Loyer E, et al. Managing synchronous liver metastases from colorectal cancer: a multidisciplinary international consensus. Cancer Treat Rev. 2015;41(9):729-41.
13. Martin J, Petrillo A, Smyth EC, Shaida N, Khwaja S, Cheow HK, et al. Colorectal liver metastases: Current management and future perspectives. World J Clin Oncol. 2020;11(10):761.
14. Fretland ÅA, Dagenborg VJ, Bjørnelv GM, Kazaryan AM, Kristiansen R, Fagerland MW, et al. Laparoscopic versus open resection for colorectal liver metastases: the OSLO-COMET randomized controlled trial. Ann Surg. 2018;267(2):199-207.
15. Adam R, Bhangui P, Poston G, Mirza D, Nuzzo G, Barroso E, et al. Is perioperative chemotherapy useful for solitary, metachronous, colorectal liver metastases?. Ann Surg. 2010;252(5):774-87.
16. Nordlinger B, Sorbye H, Glimelius B, Poston GJ, Schlag PM, Rougier P, et al. Perioperative chemotherapy with FOLFOX4 and surgery versus surgery alone for resectable liver metastases from colorectal cancer (EORTC Intergroup trial 40983): a randomised controlled trial. The Lancet. 2008;371(9617):1007-16.
17. Nordlinger B, Sorbye H, Glimelius B, Poston GJ, Schlag PM, Rougier P, et al. Perioperative FOLFOX4 chemotherapy and surgery versus surgery alone for resectable liver metastases from colorectal cancer (EORTC 40983): long-term results of a randomised, controlled, phase 3 trial. Lancet Oncol. 2013;14(12):1208-15.
18. Bonney GK, Coldham C, Adam R, Kaiser G, Barroso E, Capussotti L, et al. Role of neoadjuvant chemotherapy in resectable synchronous colorectal liver metastasis; an international multi-center data analysis using LiverMetSurvey. J Surg Oncol. 2015;111(6):716-24.

CHAPTER 7.2

Colorectal—Inflammatory Bowel Disease and Intestinal TB

■ HISTORY

History of loose stools: Patients with inflammatory bowel disease (IBD) related colitis present with frequent loose stools mixed with blood and mucus.

Differentiation between large and small bowel diarrhea
- *Large bowel diarrhea*: Frequent passage of small volume, semi-solid, non-offensive, stools mixed with blood and mucus. Note the duration of symptoms to know when the disease process began as long standing ulcerative colitis (UC) increases the risk of developing malignancy.
- *Small bowel diarrhea*: Infrequent, large volume, foul smelling, watery diarrhea
- *Presence of blood clots*: Suggests significant bleed.
- *Frequency and volume*: To gauge the blood loss.
  - Frequency of bloody stools, systemic inflammatory response syndrome (SIRS), anemia form components of Truelove and Witt's criteria of severity of UC (mentioned in the management part).
  - History of fatigue, shortness of breath, postural dizziness, syncope, need for blood transfusion: To know the severity of bleed and presence of these features points to the presence of anemia

History of associated abdominal pain: Patients with UC may have crampy left iliac fossa pain relieved by defecation.

History of urgency, tenesmus (sensation of incomplete evacuation of bowels) and nocturnal defecation which are irritative rectal symptoms: Indicative of IBD or malignancy.

History of spurious diarrhea: Colorectal cancer (seen with longstanding IBD) may lead to partial bowel obstruction, which results in the build-up of fluid and stool in the colon. This stagnant stool then liquifies, mixed with mucus proximal to the obstruction, to present as what is known as spurious diarrhea.

History of colicky abdominal pain, nausea, vomiting, abdominal distension, ball rolling sensation: Indicative of small bowel obstruction seen with Crohn's disease and ITB, due to stricturing type of disease.

History of perianal pain: Indicative of fissure in ano/abscess

History of perianal discharge: Indicative of fistula in ano/ruptured abscess

Perineal involvement in form of fissure, fistula, abscess and skin tags is more commonly seen in Crohn's colitis compared to ulcerative colitis and its presence is indicative of Crohn's disease/intestinal tuberculosis (ITB).

History of mass per rectum: Indicative of either prolapsed internal hemorrhoids, external hemorrhoids, rectal prolapse or tumor. Ask whether it is soft (benign) or firm (neoplastic), prolapsing with straining (hemorrhoids/rectal prolapse) or not, reducible (hemorrhoids/rectal prolapse) or not and whether any history of incontinence.

History of fecaluria is indicative of recto-urinary/colo-urinary fistula.

History of incontinence: If present, then sphincter saving surgery has to be avoided.

History of fever: May be seen in as a component of systemic inflammatory response syndrome (used to grade UC severity as per Truelove and Witts criteria) or it may be seen in Crohn's disease/ITB indicative of abscess/phlegmon formation due to penetrating type of disease (IBD/ITB).

History indicative of extraintestinal manifestatations of IBD
- *History of painful red/watery eyes*: Iridocyclitis
- *History of skin lesions*:
    - Erythematous, firm, solid, deep nodules or plaques that are painful on palpation and mainly localized on extensor surfaces of the legs—*erythema nodosum*
    - Painful, progressive, purple ulcers with overhanging borders on legs (most commonly pretibial)—*pyoderma gangrenosum*
- *History of joint pain*: Arthritis/ankylosing spondylitis
- *Presence of pruritus, fatigue, jaundice, ± fever*: Primary sclerosing cholangitis
- *History of weight loss, loss of appetite*: Due to SIRS or malignancy developing on the background of IBD.
- *Treatment history*: With oral/rectal tablets (mesalamine/budesonide)

History of hospital admission, ICU stay, need for surgery: Indicative of severe disease. Ask whether a stoma was created or surgeries were carried out in succession (as part of a staged procedure in UC).
- *3 staged (done for emergency indications)*: Abdominal colectomy with ileostomy → Completion proctectomy with ileal pouch anal anastomosis with diverting ileostomy → ileostoma reversal
- *2 staged*: Total proctocolectomy with ileal pouch-anal anastomosis (IPAA) with diverting ileostomy → ileostoma reversal
- *Modified 2 stage*: Abdominal colectomy with ileostomy → completion proctectomy with IPAA without diverting ileostoma
- *Single stage (done only in a fit, preserved patient in an elective setting)*: Total proctocolectomy with IPAA.

Past history:
- *History of appendectomy*: Appendectomy when done <20 years of age is considered to be protective against UC

- *History of recent travel or outside food intake*: Infective diarrhea
- *History of long-term antibiotic use*: Pseudomembranous colitis associated diarrhea due to *Clostridium difficile*.
- *History of radiation exposure*: Radiation enteritis leading to diarrhea

Personal history:
- *History of smoking*: Protective for UC but causative for Crohn's
- *If family completed or not*: If the patient is unmarried or if family is not complete then total proctectomy surgery can be deferred for preservation of fertility. If surgery cannot be deferred, then patients should be counseled regarding sperm/ovum banking.

Family history of IBD: NOD2 gene in Crohn's disease (CD) and HLA-B27 in UC.

Performance history: As per ECOG (Eastern Cooperative Oncology Group) classification to know if the patient will tolerate surgical stress or at least chemo/radiotherapy.

EXAMINATION PROFORMA

General Examination: Part A
- *Visual appearance*:
  - Young/middle aged/elderly
- *Gender*:
  - Male/female
- *Built*: Poor/average/good
- *Nourishment:* Poor/average/good
  - Measure height, weight, BMI

Clinical evaluation:
- Conscious/stuporous
- Cooperative/uncooperative
- Orientation to time, place and person: Present/absent
- Hydration status: Hydrated/dehydrated
- Lying comfortably bed/in discomfort/in pain
- Whether patient prefers sitting or lying down position
- Febrile/Afebrile

Vitals: Pulse, BP, respiratory rate, mention performance status here as well.

General Examination: Part B
Look for PICCLE, Oral cavity (aphthous ulcers), extraintestinal manifestations (EIM) [ocular, skin, joints, stigmata of chronic liver disease (CLD)]:
- *PICCLE*: Pallor, icterus (primary sclerosing cholangitis), cyanosis, clubbing, generalized or localized lymphadenopathy, palpable cervical and left supraclavicular lymph node, pedal or dependent edema
- *Examination of oral cavity*: Look for aphthous ulcers which may be seen in patients with Crohn's disease/ITB

- *Examination of eyes*: To look for iridocyclitis
- *Skin lesions*: Look for skin lesions like erythema nodosum, pyoderma gangrenosum (as already discussed above) and scratch marks (pruritus due to primary sclerosing cholangitis)
- *Joints*: Look for inflamed, erythematous, swollen joints with restricted movements indicative of arthritis/ankylosing spondylitis
- *Signs of CLD (due to long standing primary sclerosing cholangitis)*

ABDOMINAL EXAMINATION

On inspection see if:
- Abdominal contour: Flat/distended/scaphoid
- Umbilicus: Central/displaced. Inverted/everted/flat
- All quadrants are moving equally with respiration or not
- Any visible lump/nodule.

Look for:
- Visible scar, sinus, engorged veins, pulsations, peristalsis or cough impulse
- Mention scars of previous surgeries

Describe stoma:
Site:
- Right lower quadrant (ileostomy)
- Right upper quadrant (transverse colostomy)
- Left lower quadrant (sigmoidostomy)
- Single lumen (end stoma) or two lumens (loop or double barreled stoma)

Effluent: Enteric (small bowel) or fecal (colon)

Look for:
- Any mucosal lesion as in erythema, granularity, erosion or ulcer
- Prolapse
- Any skin excoriation
- Peri-stomal hernia
- Sunken stoma
- Inspect the groin hernial sites and examine genitalia.
- Inspection of renal angles to look for fullness

On palpation: See if
- Abdomen is soft, non-tender
- Liver is palpable or not (hepatomegaly may be present in case of liver metastasis)
- If palpable, measure its extent from costal margin in midclavicular line
- It is tender/nontender
- Consistency is soft/firm/hard
- Surface is smooth/nodular
- Borders are round/sharp, regular/irregular
- Margins
- Spleen is enlarged or not
- Palpate groin hernia sites and examine genitals

- Look for tenderness in renal angles
- Examine back and spine for tenderness.

On percussion:
- Look for upper border of liver dullness (generally in the 5th intercostal space) in midclavicular line
- Note the liver span (normal being 12–14 cm)
- Percussion note in the rest of the abdomen (generally tympanic)
- Tests for free fluid

On auscultation:
- Auscultate for bowel sounds. Hear for hyperperistaltic bowel sounds, for subacute intestinal obstruction (SAIO) that may result due to CD/ITB
- Auscultate for bruit, hum and rub

PER-RECTAL EXAMINATION PROFORMA

- Diaper or pad if being used
- Look for excoriation of perianal skin due to feces in a patient with incontinence or in a patient using diaper.
- Look for fissure, perianal abscess, sinus, external opening of fistula in ano, skin tag, external/internal hemorrhoids, growth or prolapse

Digital rectal examination:
- Mention tone and squeeze pressure as the first point. If the sphincter function is poor, then sphincter saving procedures should not be done.
- Assess distance of the growth (if present concomitantly) from anal verge and anal ring.
- Assess the longitudinal and circumferential extent extent of the growth
- *Consistency*: Soft/firm/hard
- *Form*: Ulcerative/proliferative/ulcero-proliferative/polypoidal
- *Fixity*: Fixed or not
- Note the staining on the gloved finger: Normal stool/blood/mucus/pus.
- Proctoscopy to complete the examination.
    - IBD → erythematous, inflamed, granular, friable mucosa with ulcers or erosion
    - Malignancy→ all the above points and its proximal and distal extent to be noted

Rest systemic examination

MANAGEMENT

Ulcerative Colitis

Truelove and Witts criteria for Severity of Ulcerative Colitis
- *Frequency of bloody stools*:
    - Mild: ≤4 stools/day with or without blood
    - Moderate: 4–6 stools/day with blood
    - Severe: > 6 bloody stools/day

- *Fever*:
  - Mild: < 37.5°C
  - Moderate: 37.5–37.8°C
  - Severe: > 37.8°C
- *Pulse*:
  - Mild: < 90 bpm
  - Moderate: ≤90 bpm
  - Severe: > 90 bpm
- *Hemoglobin*:
  - Mild: > 11.5 g/dL
  - Moderate: 10.5–11.5 g/dL
  - Severe: < 10.5 g/dL.
- *Erythrocyte sedimentation rate (ESR)*:
  - Mild: < 20 mm/h
  - Moderate: 20–30 mm/h
  - Severe: > 30 mm/h

Montreal Classification for Ulcerative Colitis

- *Extent of colitis*:
  - E1: Ulcerative proctitis—limited to rectum; proximal extent being rectosigmoid junction
  - E2: Left sided colitis—disease limited to the left colon: proximal extent being splenic flexure.
  - E3: Extensive colitis—disease extends proximal to the splenic flexure. It includes pancolitis and backwash ileitis.
- *Severity of disease*:
  - S0: Clinical remission
  - S1: Mild disease as per Truelove and Witts criteria (discussed previously)
  - S2: Moderate disease as per Truelove and Witts criteria
  - S3: Severe disease as per Truelove and Witts criteria

Treatment of Mild-to-moderate Ulcerative Colitis[1]

5 aminosalicylic acid (ASA) (oral 2–4.8 g/day and rectal 1–2 g/day), if no response, then budesonide (rectal 0.2 mg/day) OR budesonide multimatrix formulation (MMX) for left/extensive (oral 9 mg/day), if no response, oral steroids (0.75–1 mg/kg/day) and then it can either respond to this treatment, or present as the following.

Steroid-refractory Ulcerative Colitis

- Patients not responding to steroid treatment with 0.75–1 mg/kg/day of oral prednisolone/equivalent within 4 weeks or IV for at least 1 week, after infectious complications (CMV, *C. difficile*-associated disease) have been excluded, are defined to have steroid-refractory UC.
- In active steroid-refractory UC, anti-TNF (biologicals), vedolizumab (anti-integrin), tacrolimus (calcineurin inhibitor) have been shown to achieve steroid-free remission.

- If anti-TNF therapy or tacrolimus is started, combination and long-term maintenance with azathioprine/mercaptopurine (AZA/6-MP) (immunomodulators) is preferred.
- Tofacitinib (Janus kinase inhibitor) will be an option in patients with treatment failure to immunomodulators

Steroid-dependent Ulcerative Colitis

Initially responds to oral steroids but failure to taper below the equivalent of prednisolone 10 mg/day within 3 months or that relapses within 3 months after steroid discontinuation. Steroid use in UC is associated with higher risk for relapse and colectomy.

AZA/6-MP maintenance therapy is best suited for patients with low risk of progression who responded well to a first course of steroid treatment.

In all others, anti-TNF alone or in combination with AZA/6-MP, vedolizumab, or tofacitinib.

Jalan's Criteria for Toxic Megacolon

Radiographic evidence of colonic distension (>6 cm):
- *PLUS ≥3:*
  - Fever >38°C
  - Heart rate >120 beats/min
  - Anemia
  - Neutrophilic leukocytosis >10,500/microL
- *PLUS ≥1:*
  - Dehydration
  - Electrolyte disturbances
  - Hypotension
  - Altered sensorium

Management of Acute Severe Ulcerative Colitis (ASUC) and Toxic Megacolon (TMC)[1]

Preliminary Treatment

- Hydration, IV antibiotics
- Early enteral nutrition
- Rule out CMV, *C. difficile*, TB
- Give LMWH 40 mg/day

Intensive Medical Treatment

- IV prednisolone 0.8–1 mg/kg/day for 3 days, maximum 125 mg/day
- If no response after 3 days: IV infliximab (5 mg/kg/day) (if response seen, then at 2, 6 and every 8 weeks), or
- IV cyclosporine (2–4 mg/kg/day) (if response seen then oral for 3 months, with AZA and maintain with AZA/6-MP)
- If no response after 3 days, then shift for surgery.

Surgical Indications

- Steroid refractory and steroid dependent UC
- ASUC and TMC refractory to medical management

- Severe bleed, obstruction, perforation
- Cancer

Histology of UC: Crypt distortion, crypt abscess, increased lymphocytes in lamina propria, hypertrophy of muscularis mucosa and disease generally confined to mucosa.

Histology of CD: Noncaseating microgranulomas (<200 microns), while TB has caseating necrosis with macro granulomas.

IBD surveillance for cancer: After 8 years of pan colitis, random 4 quadrant biopsy, every 5 cm on left and every 10 cm on right, total 32 biopsies.

Incidence of CRC: 0.5/1,000 person-years-duration (UC > Crohn's), cumulative risk of CRC with UC: 2%, 8%, 18% after 10, 20, and 30 years.

Risk factors: Family history, PSC, left colitis (4 times risk), Pancolitis (19 times risk).

IBD with Cancer:
- Focus on treatment of cancer. Reduce/Stop anti-TNF and AZA/6-MP. Chemo helps IBD remission.
- If IBD not responding: 5 ASA, steroids—1st line. Anti-TNF—2nd line.

PSC-IBD:
- High risk for CRC and scopy within normal limits (WNL) even in active IBD.
- 70% PSC have IBD (UC is most common)
- Only 5% UC get PSC

Screening:
- In a known case of PSC—Ileocolonoscopy and random biopsy at diagnosis.
- If dysplasia/CRC manage it accordingly.
- If no IBD, repeat every 3–5 years.
- If present, then it is PSC-IBD.

Surveillance in IBD for PSC: Annual LFT, and if abnormal, do MRCP: PSC-IBD. Do viral and autoimmune panel to rule other differentials out.

Colectomy is protective for PSC, with reduced risk for future liver transplant and mortality, and reduced risk for recurrence after transplant.

Crohn's Disease

Montreal Classification for Crohn's Disease

Age of onset:
- *A1*: < 17 years
- *A2*: 17–40 years
- *A3*: > 40 years

Location:
- *L1*: Terminal ileum with or without cecum
- *L2*: Colon
- *L3*: Ileum plus colon
- *L4*: Upper GI

Behavior:
- *B1*: Nonstructuring nonpenetrating
- *B2*: Stricturing
- *B3*: Penetrating

p for perianal disease modifier

Free perforation: 1% of CD in adults, risk factors: >30 years at CD diagnosis, on steroids and anti-TNF, and presence of stricture

Enterocutaneous fistula: seen in 30% of CD.
- *Pathophysiology of penetrating disease*: Contained perforation → abscess → internal/external fistulae
- Treatment: Ciplox + Adalimumab

Surgical indications in CD:
- Long segment (≤40 cm) inflammatory type ileocolonic CD not responding to conventional treatment (LIRIC trial). Also, upfront surgery for stenosing CD (strictureplasty/resection). Remember that for small bowel, strictureplasty is favored over resection, however for colon, resection only must be done
- Toxic megacolon, refractory to medical management, bleeding, obstruction, perforation, abscess (delayed surgery after 2 weeks better), symptomatic and enterovesical/vaginal fistulae
- Perianal abscess and fistulae (PISA trial: For high fistulae, surgery + anti-TNF better than Seton + anti-TNF)
- Cancer

Surgery for CD: Minimal access better. For open, take transverse incisions, strictureplasty best except in colon where direct resection is to be done. Side-to-side anastomosis better.

Management of perianal CD:
- *Evaluation:* EUS, MRI(best), EUA.
- *Simple fistulas*: Low, below dentate, single opening, no perianal complications.
- *Complex*: High, multiple, local abscess/stricture, associated with bladder vagina.
- *St James hospital, Garg classifications.*
- *Other perianal CD*: Ulceration, stenosis, neoplasms

Treatment of CD fistulas: Drain all abscesses first. Then:
- Ciplox (1–1.5 g), Metro (0.75–1 g)/day, 8–12 weeks or Aza/6-MP >12 weeks for effect or anti-TNF-α for induction and maintenance. Combination of Ciplox and anti-TNF best, with loose setons.
- Advancement flaps, ligation of intersphincteric fistula tract (LIFT), laser, video-assisted anal fistula treatment (VAAFT) also used

Crohn's Disease versus Intestinal Tuberculosis

Clinical features of both diseases include fever, anorexia, colicky abdominal pain (biologics worsen obstruction in fibrostenotic CD), recurrent SAIO, chronic diarrhea, hematochezia, weight loss, perianal disease, and extra-intestinal manifestations (EIMs) including aphthous ulcers, ocular, dermatologic and arthralgia.

As per the latest meta-analysis by Limsrivillai et al.:[2]

Among the clinical features, presence of diarrhea, hematochezia, perianal disease, and EIMs and longer disease duration favors the diagnosis of CD, whereas presence of fever, night sweats, lung involvement and ascites favors the diagnosis of ITB.

Among the endoscopic features, the presence of recto-sigmoid involvement, longitudinal ulcers, aphthous ulcers, cobblestone appearance, mucosal bridge, luminal stricture, and skip lesions favored CD, whereas the presence of IC valve and cecal involvement, patulous IC valve and transverse ulcers favored ITB.

Among pathologic features, granulomas in CD are usually small (microgranuloma), discrete, ill-defined and sparse. Tubercular granulomas are usually large (> 200 microns), confluent, dense (> 5–10/hpf), located in submucosa, and are characterized by central caseation, which is diagnostic and exclusive for ITB. Granulomas in the surrounding lymph nodes can be seen in both diseases, but lymph nodal granulomas in the absence of intestinal inflammation are seen only in ITB.

Among the microbiologic tests, acid-fast bacteria (AFB) stain, AFB culture (Lowenstein Jensen medium, BACTEC), and gene-Xpert MTB are diagnostic for ITB, however, these tests are associated with very poor diagnostic sensitivity.

In recent study from India,[3] *CT findings* that were more common in patients with CD as compared to ITB were involvement of the left colonic segment (22% vs. 6%), long-segment involvement (69% vs. 28%), presence of skip lesions (63% vs. 42%), and presence of comb sign (44% vs. 20%). Fat hypertrophy, creeping fat and fat wrapping have been associated with active CD, and visceral fat has been correlated with disease outcomes in patients with CD.

On the other hand, the involvement of ileocecal area, shorter length of involvement, and presence of lymph nodes larger than 1 cm are more common in ITB. Addition of CT chest doubles the sensitivity of ITB diagnosis from 25 to 51%. Therefore, CT chest and CT enterography, both are recommended in the diagnostic evaluation of a patient with ulcero-constrictive intestinal disease, as evidence of active TB on CT chest will clearly tilt the diagnosis toward ITB.[4]

Positive serology for anti-saccharomyces cerevisiae antibody (ASCA) has no role in differentiating CD from ITB, as shown in two studies from India and in recent meta-analyses, where ASCA was not found useful and in 1 of the meta-analysis, the diagnostic accuracy of ASCA was only 57%.[5]

Also, both Interferon-Gamma Release Assay (IGRA) and Mantoux are predictive of latent TB rather than active TB, which practically renders them useless.

Therapeutic Antitubercular Trial

Recent Asia-Pacific consensus statements for CD have also mentioned, that in a patient with CD/ITB dilemma, the diagnosis of CD should only be considered in a patient who doesn't respond to ATT, and subsequently responds to CD-specific therapy.[6] The clinical response should be assessed at 2–3 months of ATT. In patients who are responding, ATT should be continued till 6 months, and at 6 months, a repeat endoscopy should be done to document mucosal healing. Diagnosis of ITB is confirmed in the presence of clinical and endoscopic response. In the presence of no response/worsening on ATT at 2–3 months, a repeat endoscopic/radiological evaluation should be done, and in the presence of active disease, the diagnosis of CD should be considered. Multidrug resistant tuberculosis (MDR-TB) also behaves like CD when considering clinical/endoscopic/radiologic non-response to ATT. However, ITB is a paucibacillary disease, and studies from South Korea and India have shown low prevalence (< 5%) of MDR-TB among patients with ITB.[7,8]

However, in the presence of diagnostic features of ITB, and non-response to ATT, the possibility of MDR-TB should be considered.[9]

Remember three factors which have 100% specificity in differentiating ITB from Crohn's:
1. Necrotic lymph node on CT
2. Caseation necrosis on biopsy
3. Positive acid-fast bacillus smear/culture

These three are the only differentiating features with 100% specificity, though are limited by poor sensitivity.[9]

Medical Management

Primary Modality of Treatment

As per the RNTCP act, it consists of administration of category 1 anti-tuberculosis therapy (ATT): Isoniazid (H), rifampicin (R), pyrazinamide (Z) and ethambutol (E) in daily dosages as per 4 weight band categories for 6 months (intensive phase—2 months and continuation phase 4 months).

In case of relapse, treatment failure or treatment defaulter, category two ATT- H, R, Z, E, and streptomycin (S) is administered.

Indications for Surgery

- Obstruction
- Phlegmon/abscess
- Perforation
- Internal or external fistula
- Diagnostic dilemma (ileocaecal mass as TB vs. Crohn's vs. cancer)

ATT needs to be initiated in the postoperative period.

REFERENCES

1. Burri E, Maillard MH, Schoepfer AM, Seibold F, Van Assche G, Rivière P, Laharie D, Manz M. Treatment algorithm for mild and moderate-to-severe ulcerative colitis: an update. Digestion. 2020 Sep 29;101(Suppl. 1):2-15.
2. Limsrivilai J, Shreiner AB, Pongpaibul A, Laohapand C, Boonanuwat R, Pausawasdi N, et al. Meta-analytic Bayesian model for differentiating intestinal tuberculosis from Crohn's disease. Am J Gastroenterol. 2017;112(3):415-27.
3. Kedia S, Sharma R, Nagi B, Mouli VP, Aananthakrishnan A, Dhingra R, et al. Computerized tomography-based predictive model for differentiation of Crohn's disease from intestinal tuberculosis. Indian J Gastroenterol. 2015;34:135-43.
4. Almadi MA, Ghosh S, Aljebreen AM. Differentiating intestinal tuberculosis from Crohn's disease: a diagnostic challenge. Am J Gastroenterol. 2009;104(4):1003-12.
5. Ng SC, Hirai HW, Tsoi KK, Wong SH, Chan FK, Sung JJ, et al. Systematic review with meta-analysis: Accuracy of interferon-gamma releasing assay and anti-S accharomyces cerevisiae antibody in differentiating intestinal tuberculosis from C rohn's disease in A sians. J Gastroenterol Hepatol. 2014;29(9):1664-70.
6. Ooi CJ, Makharia GK, Hilmi I, Gibson PR, Fock KM, Ahuja V, et al. Asia Pacific Consensus Statements on Crohn's disease. Part 1: Definition, diagnosis, and epidemiology: (Asia Pacific Crohn's Disease Consensus—Part 1). J Gastroenterol Hepatol. 2016;31(1):45-55.
7. Ye BD, Yang SK, Kim D, Shim TS, Kim SH, Kim MN, et al. Diagnostic sensitivity of culture and drug resistance patterns in Korean patients with intestinal tuberculosis. Int J Tuberc Lung Dis. 2012;16(6):799-804.
8. Samant H, Desai D, Abraham P, Joshi A, Gupta T, Rodrigues C, et al. Acid-fast bacilli culture positivity and drug resistance in abdominal tuberculosis in Mumbai, India. Indian J Gastroenterol. 2014;33:414-9.
9. Almadi MA, Ghosh S, Aljebreen AM. Differentiating intestinal tuberculosis from Crohn's disease: a diagnostic challenge. Am J Gastroenterol. 2009;104(4):1003-12.

7.3 CHAPTER

Colorectal—Ward

Nerve injury during TME can occur at four points:
1. During high ligation of inferior mesenteric artery (IMA) [superior hypogastric plexus (SHP): sympathetic supply. Can lead to incontinence and retrograde ejaculation]
   At sacral promontory, SHP again.
2. During lateral pelvic side wall lymph node (LN) dissection (only if present on MRI), can damage parasympathetic nerve supply. Can lead to bladder atony and erectile dysfunction
3. At the level of seminal vesicles/dome of bladder, inferior hypogastric plexus (IHP). Contains sympathetic and parasympathetic supply. Can lead to above both symptoms.
4. Also at level of lateral stalks, IHP may get damaged.

Suppose if specimen of total proctocolectomy (TPC) for inflammatory bowel disease (IBD)/familial adenomatous polyposis (FAP) shows distal rectal malignancy, with free margins, involved nodes then consider adjuvant chemo RT (radiotherapy) (5-FU or Capecitabine based CRT, 50 Gy:1.8 Gy/day) *for 6 months*.

The ESMO recommends it for any tumor ≥T3b, node positive, CRM+, tumor perforation, for which neoadjuvant treatment has not been given. Adjuvant RT alone is obsolete.

Suppose if distal margin of specimen comes positive for cancer, then counsel patient regarding resurgery versus adjuvant CRT. If young then resurgery preferred, so, then if initial procedure was anterior resection (AR), do low anterior resection (LAR) and if LAR then do ultra low anterior resection (ULAR), and if ULAR, then do intersphincteric resection (ISR), and if ISR, then go for abdominoperineal resection (APR). However, if elderly, then better to go for adjuvant CRT (5-FU or Capecitabine based RT).

APR indication: T4/low rectal cancer invading intersphincteric space/external anal sphincter/pelvic floor, recurrent rectal cancer, salvage treatment for anal cancer, refractory anorectal CD.

Perineal approach: Elliptical incision.

Anteriorly: Perineal body, Posteriorly: Coccyx, Bilaterally: Ischial tuberosity. Division of anococcygeal raphe, ilio and ischiococcygeal muscles, and levators at dentate.

APR versus extralevator abdominoperineal excision (ELAPE):
- *Position*: Supine(S) in APR versus S+/-Prone in ELAPE.
- CRM+, perforation rates high in APR.
- Wound issues in ELAPE.

CHAPTER 8

Lump in Abdomen

Lump in abdomen as a case is a tricky prospect, however, to make it simpler, as you go taking history, think quadrant and organ-wise and ask questions relevant to the pathologies arising from each organ/system in that specific quadrant. And when history and examination of the lump are complete, and if the clinical picture is more or less suggestive of a benign lesion, then formulate your differentials accordingly; do not force malignancies into your list. And vice versa.

The following is the quadrant-wise distribution of organs giving the first clue from where the pathology may be originating:

▪ EPIGASTRIUM

- Biliary
- Left lobe of liver
- Stomach
- Transverse colon
- Body of pancreas
- Retroperitoneum

▪ RIGHT UPPER QUADRANT

- Liver
- Gallbladder
- Distal stomach
- Head of pancreas
- Distal ascending, hepatic flexure of colon and proximal transverse colon
- Right adrenal and kidney
- Retroperitoneum

▪ RIGHT LOWER QUADRANT

- Terminal ileum
- Cecum

- Ascending colon
- Appendix
- Mesentery

LEFT UPPER QUADRANT

- Spleen
- Splenic flexure of colon
- Distal transverse and proximal descending colon
- Tail of pancreas
- Body of stomach left kidney and adrenal retroperitoneum
- Left lower quadrant
- Descending and sigmoid colon

COMMON TO BOTH LOWER QUADRANTS

- Kidney lower pole
- Ectopic kidney
- Undescended testis tubo-ovarian structures
- Retroperitoneum

So the clinically important pathologies arising from the above mentioned organ/systems are discussed below:

LIVER LESIONS

Hepatic Adenoma

Generally asymptomatic. Seen more commonly in females secondary to OCP use. Males on anabolic steroids can also land up with hepatic adenomas. Hepatic adenomatosis can occur in glycogen storage disorders and maturity-onset diabetes of the young (MODY). Adenomas may rupture and cause severe abdominal pain and even hemoperitoneum and can even turn malignant (especially the beta catenin variant).

On palpation a firm, non-tender lump, continuous with the liver, may be felt in the RUQ which moves with respiration.

On auscultation over a large peripheral adenoma, vascular bruit may be heard.

Focal Nodular Hyperplasia

Considered as a differential in a young female with lump in RUQ. Has no predisposing factors/history. Abdominal examination findings similar to the above. However, remember that FNH is most often a radiological diagnosis and nothing more needs to be done. However, in case of a diagnostic dilemma, surgical resection is often performed and then the diagnosis is known only in the postoperative HPE.

Hepatic Hemangioma
- Again, has no predisposing factors/history. Generally asymptomatic. An atypical/giant hemangioma (>10 cm), may present with dragging type of pain in RUQ. Consumptive coagulopathy and congestive heart failure may be seen in infants with Kasabach–Merritt syndrome. Bornman–Terblanche–Blumgart syndrome, may present with a palpable atypical/giant hemangioma along with fever (inflammatory syndrome).
- Abdominal examination findings similar to the above.
- On auscultation vascular bruit may be heard over a large hemangioma.

Hepatocellular Carcinoma (HCC)
Management already discussed in the Chapter 3.3.

Ask for: History indicative of cirrhosis as HCC develops on a background of cirrhosis. However, remember that HBV can lead to HCC even without cirrhosis (due to insertional mutagenesis) while fibrolamellar HCC presents in a non-cirrhotic liver and has none of the etiological factors of conventional HCC.

History indicative of cirrhosis:
- Abdominal distension (ascites)
- Icterus, Jaundice (liver cell failure)
- GI bleed (variceal bleed)
- Altered sensorium (hepatic encephalopathy)
- Reduced urine output (hepatorenal syndrome)

History to suggest symptomatic hypersplenism (portal hypertension): Anemia, petechiae, infections.

History of alcohol consumption (to rule out ethanol related cirrhosis), history of recurring jaundice, previous blood transfusion, high risk sexual behavior, IV drug abuse (to rule out all etiologies of viral hepatitis B, C leading to cirrhosis).

History of loss of weight; loss of appetite: Alarming pointers toward malignancy.

History of metastatic disease:
- *Abdominal distension*: Due to malignant ascites
- *Dry cough, hemoptysis*: Due to pleural effusion and lung metastasis
- *Bony pain, non-traumatic fractures*: Due to bony metastasis
- *Back pain*: Due to vertebral metastasis
- *Unexplained sudden new onset headaches, blackouts, seizures*: Due to brain metastasis
- On examination look for icterus, and signs of CLD and portal hypertension (abdominal distension, dilated engorged paraumbilical veins and splenomegaly)
- Abdominal examination findings similar to the above.

Hepatic Metastasis

If history is suggestive of malignancy developing in GI system/pasthistory of treatment for any other site primary, along with palpable liver lesions/hepatomegaly then keep liver metastases in your differentials.

Cystic liver lesions can be infective or non-infective.
Infective: Amebic liver abscess (ALA), pyogenic liver abscess (PLA), fungal abscess and hydatid cyst.

Non-infective:
- *Benign*: Simple cyst, polycystic liver disease (PCLD), biliary hamartoma (Von Meyenburg complex)
- *Premalignant*: Choledochal cyst (CDC), Caroli's, mucinous cystic neoplasm-liver (MCN-L), intraductal papillary mucinous neoplasm-Biliary (IPMN-B)
- *Malignant*: Cystic metastases (from CRC/ovarian), cystic HCC, cystic NET, biliary cystadenocarcinoma (BCAC)
- *Traumatic*: Biloma, seroma, hematoma

Hepatic Abscess

There will be history of RUQ abdominal pain, fever, chills. There may be jaundice. Amebic liver abscess usually develops in young alcoholic males, and history of colitis/diarrhea may be present concomitantly, though not always. Pyogenic abscess commonly develops in the elderly secondary to biliary block-malignant obstructive jaundice and in the young due to biliary calculi; or secondary to diverticulitis (left lower quadrant abdominal pain, fever, GI bleed) appendicitis, leading to portal venous pyemia and liver abscess. Fungal abscess develops in patients with prolonged exposure to antibiotics, hematologic malignancies, solid-organ transplants, and congenital and acquired immunodeficiency, including those with diabetes mellitus, on high dose steroids, etc., with similar presentation.

On examination, tender lump in the RUQ/epigastrium which is continuous with the liver, going under the rib cage, which moves with respiration, will be palpable.

Hydatid Cyst

Seen in endemic areas where sheep grazing, cattle grazing, shepherding, animal husbandry are the main occupations. History of contact with a pet animal could be present. There are two main forms of hydatidosis—the cystic echinococcosis form and the alveolar echinococcosis form.

Cystic Echinococcosis (CE) (Tables 1 and 2)

Caused by the parasite, *Echinococcus granulosus* a cestode that lives in the small intestine of dogs and other canines.

Patient may be asymptomatic, or may have RUQ abdominal pain/discomfort/heaviness. Fever if present is indicative of secondary cyst infection. In case of cysto-biliary communication (generally cysts present at the hilum/compressing

TABLE 1: Ultrasonography classification of echinococcal cyst. WHO classification of cystic echinococcosis.[1]

WHO IWGE 2001	Image	Description	Stage
CE1		Unilocular, anechoic cyst with double line sign	Active
CE2		Multiseptate honeycomb cyst	
CE3a		Cyst with detached membranes	Transitional
CE3b		Cyst with daughter cysts in solid matrix	
CE4		Cyst with heterogeneous hypoechoic/hyperechoic contents. No daughter cysts	Inactive
CE5		Solid plus calcified wall	

TABLE 2: Management as per WHO classification.[2]

Treatment modalities stratified by cyst stage (uncompliacted)

WHO classification	Suggested practice
CE1	Albendazole alone if < 5 cm PAIR + Albendazole if > 5 cm
CE2	Surgery + Albendazole Or Non-PAIR PT + Albendazole
CE3a	Albendazole alone if < 5 cm PAIR + Albendazole if > 5 cm
CE3b	Surgery + Albendazole Non-PAIR PT + Albendazole
CE4 and 5	Wait and watch

large ducts, present with this) patient will present with jaundice, may develop cholangitis (Charcot's triad: Pain, fever and jaundice) and hence doing an MRCP for large cysts is absolutely essential before taking up the patient for surgery. Rupture into the peritoneal cavity seeding daughter cysts, may lead to anaphylaxis or disseminated hydatidosis in the peritoneal cavity, whereas intrathoracic rupture/spread via blood stream may lead to lung dissemination and may even present as coughing out of hydatid content.

On palpation a firm, rounded, tender/non-tender lump may be felt in the RUQ which is continuous with the liver, going under the rib cage, which moves with respiration. Hydatid thrill may be present (WHO types 1–3).

However, CE4 and CE5 cysts if symptomatic—causing pain/jaundice due to compression, must be operated to relieve the symptoms.

Conservative procedures aim at sterilization and evacuation of cyst content, including the hydatid membrane (hydatidectomy), and partial removal of the cyst. The evacuation and hydatidectomy consists of cyst puncture and aspiration of part of the contents for introduction of scolicidal agent, allowing contact time (20% hypertonic saline is recommended with a contact with the germinal layer for at least 15 minutes), and total aspiration following that.

After partial removal of the cyst, residual cavity may get secondarily infected leading to abscess formation or it may lead to formation of biloma due to Cystobiliary communications (CBCs) which were not/could not be addressed. The residual cavities are thus managed by simple drainage with suction and filling with omentum (omentoplasty) to reduce the risk of complications.

Radical procedures aim at complete removal of the cyst with or without hepatic resection, have greater intraoperative risks and postoperative complications, but lower relapses.

For prevention of relapses—Albendazole should be given 10–15 mg/kg body weight in two divided doses daily, starting 1 week before surgery and continuing to up to at least 3 months after surgery.

How to Diagnose and Manage Cystobiliary Communication on the Table
Firstly, aspirate the cyst with a small needle, see the color. If frankly bilious, that is a clinical pointer to CBC. If facilities are available, send it to the lab for analysis for bilirubin. If it is >3 times the serum value, that confirms the suspicion. Another method is to inject methylene blue into the biliary system, temporarily clamp the CBD distally and then if staining is present in the cystic fluid, CBC is present.
- So if CBC is present, aspirate the cyst contents completely, then deroof the cyst.
- *Do not* inject any scolicidal agent at it may lead to chemical cholangitis and biliary strictures.
- Visually see the places where CBC is present and suture it with 4–0 PDS. Check if the bile leak has stopped by again performing the above steps.
- In case of a large calibre duct communicating with the cyst, biliary-enteric anastomosis or liver resection are sometimes necessary.
- Presence of CBC also leads to passage of cyst fluid and contents into the CBD. If ERCP and CBD clearance is not achieved preoperatively, then do a choledochotomy, clear the CBD, and after administering IV glucagon (to relax the sphincter of Oddi), flush the CBD liberally with saline and ensure complete clearance with choledochoscope.

Laparoscopic Approach in the Management of Hydatid Cyst and CBC
Concerns of laparoscopic management of hydatid cyst:
- Spillage
- Incomplete evacuation of cystic contents

Many devices devised to prevent spillage and to enable complete evacuation of the hydatid cyst:
- Professor Palanivelu's "Palanivelu Hydatid System" (PHS) consists of a complex system of fenestrated trocar and cannulas which helps in:
  - Preventing spillage
  - Complete evacuation of contents and allows
  - Intracystic magnified view of cyst-biliary communication for repair

For lung hydatid, Albendazole should be avoided preoperatively in large cysts. Surgery should be as conservative as possible.

Alveolar Echinococcosis (AE) (Table 3)
Caused by the parasite, *Echinococcus multilocularis*. Patient may again be asymptomatic, or may have RUQ abdominal pain/discomfort/heaviness.

On palpation a firm, rounded, non-tender lump may be felt in the RUQ which is continuous with the liver, going under the rib cage, which moves with respiration.

Alveolar echinococcosis is a malignant form of a relatively benign disease, which presents as a solid-cystic form of hydatidosis. Serological tests may help differentiate between cystic and alveolar echinococcosis. The use of *E. multilocularis* antigens (Em2, Em2+, Em18) has a high diagnostic sensitivity

TABLE 3: WHO-IWGE PNM classification of alveolar echinococcosis.

PNM classification of alveolar echinococcosis	
P	Hepatic localization of the parasite
PX	Primary tumor cannot be assessed
P0	No detectable tumor in the liver
P1	Peripheral lesions without proximal vascular and/or biliary involvement
P2	Central lesions with proximal vascular and/or biliary involvement of one lobe[a]
P3	Central lesions with hilar vascular or biliary involvement of both lobes and/or with involvement of two hepatic veins
P4	Any liver lesion with extension along the vessels[b] and the biliary tree
N	Extrahepatic involvement of neighboring organs [diaphragm, lung, pleura, pericardium, heart, gastric and duodenal wall, adrenal glands, peritoneum, retroperitoneum, parietal wall (muscles, skin, bone), pancreas, regional lymph nodes, liver ligaments, kidney]
NX	Not evaluable
N0	No regional involvement
N1	Regional involvement of contiguous organs or tissues
M	The absence or presence of distant metastasis (lung, distant lymph nodes, spleen, CNS, orbital, bone, skin, muscle, kidney, distant peritoneum and retroperitoneum)
MX	Not completely evaluated
M0	No metastasis[c]
M1	Metastasis

[a] For classification, the plane projecting between the bed of the gallbladder and the inferior vena cava divides the liver into two lobes.
[b] Vessels mean inferior vena cava, portal vein, and arteries.
[c] Chest X-ray and cerebral CT negative.
Source: WHO/OIE, 2001; Kern et al., 2006.

and specificity of 90–100%, which allows discrimination between AE and CE in 80–95% of cases. (WHO-IWGE, 1996; WHO/OIE, 2001; Ito and Craig, 2003). However, triphasic liver protocol CECT is generally characteristic showing pseudocystic areas due to large areas of central necrosis and the typical pattern of calcification. MR imaging may show the multivesicular morphology of the lesions. In diagnostic dilemma, biopsy of the lesion confirms the diagnosis.

This disease literally eats into the liver and when patients finally present, the imaging reveals multiple sections involved as a result of which major hepatectomy (≥3 sections) is often required (2 cm safety margin recommended—Marchiondo et al., 1994; Sato et al., 1997; Uchino et al., 1993), and the patient may even be deemed inoperable due to inadequate FLR, for which liver transplant remains the only salvage (however, postoperative immunosuppression may lead to disease relapse).

Albendazole should be given for at least 2 years and these patients monitored for a minimum of 10 years for possible recurrence (Reuter et al., 2000).

For Albendazole toxicity—monitor weekly, monthly and then every 3 monthly with CBC and LFT.
- If AST/ALT deranged, decrease the dosage
- If leukocyte count goes under 1.0×10^9/L, stop the treatment till the counts recover

Simple Hepatic Cyst

Generally asymptomatic. Pain can result due to liver capsular stretch/bleeding into the cyst, whereas, if the cyst gets secondarily infected, it can present with fever.

A large cyst can lead to a nontender soft/firm (tense cystic) palpable lump in the RUQ/epigastrium which is continuous with the liver, going under the rib cage, which moves with respiration.

Polycystic Liver Disease (PCLD)
- Similar findings as simple hepatic cyst, may present with multiple renal cysts.
- Schnelldorfer classification is used to classify the cystic burden and management which depends upon number of uninvolved sections of liver and whether vascular occlusion is present in those sections **(Table 4)**

TABLE 4: Schnelldorfer classification.[3]

	Type A	Type B	Type C	Type D
Symptoms	Absent or mild	Moderate or severe	Severe (or moderate)	Severe (or moderate)
Cyst characteristics	Any	Limited number of large cysts	Any	Any
Areas of relative normal liver parenchyma	Any	≥2 sections	≥1 section	<1 section
Presence of portal vein or hepatic vein occlusion in the preserved hepatic sections	Any	Absent	Absent	Present
Recommended therapy	Observation or medical therapy	Cyst fenestration	Partial hepatectomy with possible fenestration of remnant cysts	Liver transplantation

Mucinous Neoplasms of the Liver

World Health Organization (WHO) classified mucin-producing bile duct tumors of the liver as two distinct entities: Mucinous cystic neoplasm of the liver (MCN-L) and intraductal papillary mucinous neoplasm of the bile duct (IPMN-B).

Mucinous Cystic Neoplasm of the Liver
- Histologically differentiated from IPMN-B based on mucin-producing epithelium associated with ovarian-like stroma (OLS)
- Mostly often located in segment 4 of liver and are generally solitary
- Having a female predisposition

Intraductal Papillary Mucinous Neoplasm of the Bile Duct
- Differentiated from MCN-L by the lack of OLS and the presence of communication with the bile ducts. Copious amount of mucin produced resulting in grossly dilated bile ducts. May be multicentric and thus complete cholangioscopic examination must be done before definitive surgery.
- Biliary counterpart of intraductal papillary mucinous neoplasm of the pancreas (IPMN-P)
- *Classified into four subtypes based on tumor cells*: Gastric, intestinal, pancreaticobiliary and oncocytic

R0 resection of MCN-L and IPMN-B both have a good prognosis, but resection of MCN-L has an even better survival than IPMN-B (probably due to the multicentricity, and the presence of aggressive types like pancreaticobiliary).

R0 resection of MCN-L is generally curative, however, IPMN-B requires 6 monthly follow-up just like IPMN-P.

Malignant Liver Cystic Primaries
BCAC and even HCC, NET may present in a cystic form and the abdominal examination findings are same as for the other liver SOLs mentioned above, except there is no tenderness on palpation.

Hepatic Cystic Metastasis
Metastases from CRC/ovarian cancer may present in a cystic form and the abdominal examination findings are same as for the other liver SOLs mentioned above, except there is no tenderness on palpation.

Biloma
Patients with bile duct injury may present in the immediate postoperative period with a biloma in case the external biliary fistula is not controlled or in the postoperative period following any HPB surgery if the drains are not draining the bilary leak completely. Also, patients with blunt abdominal trauma with liver injuries managed conservatively may present with biloma resulting from bile leak.

Management
- Image guided percutaneous drain (PCD) placement, and at times multiple PCDs may be needed to drain the collection
- If inspite of multiple PCDs, there are still pockets of undrained/loculated collection/the patient continues to be in sepsis due to inadequate source

control, then laparoscopic copius lavage with normal saline and placement of drains must be done.

GALLBLADDER

Mucocele
RUQ/Epigastric pain +– radiating to right infrascapular region, worsening postprandially. Distended nontender GB will be palpable in the RUQ.

Empyema
Patient will have a toxic look, with history of pain, fever, chills. Distended tender GB will be palpable. However, diabetics may have empyema and even emphysematous cholecystitis with minimal symptoms and signs so beware of callousness.

Xanthogranulomatous Cholecystitis
Is actually a postoperative pathological diagnosis, as preoperatively it is almost impossible to differentiate between XGC and gallbladder cancer (GBC). Thus all GB masses especially in high GBC incidence areas must be treated as GBC until proven as XGC on postoperative HPE. However clinically, patient will give history of multiple attacks of biliary colic, fever and maybe even jaundice if the disease extends into the biliary tree. There will not be loss of weight and loss of appetite. Firm to hard mass will be palpable in the RHC.

GBC: Has already been discussed in detail (Chapter 3)
Again past history of cholecystitis may be present. GBC neck presents early as jaundice along with pruritus, whereas GBC body/fundus infiltrating liver may present with a palpable hard mass and with pain of liver infiltration, while GBC body/fundus infiltrating stomach/duodenum may present with gastric outlet obstruction (GOO) and GI bleed.

Distal blocks (Periampullary malignancy, carcinoma head of pancreas, distal cholangiocarcinoma) and also GBC neck occluding cystic duct—leading to distended palpable GB, this GB is nontender and soft. However, keep in mind that a grossly distended, tense cystic GB, will be firm to palpate even when the pathology is not in the GB wall per se.

COLONIC LESION: Has already been discussed in detail (Chapter 7)

GASTRIC LESION: Has already been discussed in detail (Chapter 2)

Distal body/antropyloric malignancy:
- Adenocarcinoma
- Lymphoma
- GIST

PANCREATIC LESION: Has already been discussed in detail (Chapter 3)

- *Pancreatic neoplasms*:
  - Adenocarcinoma, NET
  - Cystic lesions—serous cystadenoma, MCN, IPMN
  - Pancreatic pseudocyst

SPLENOMEGALY COMMON CAUSES WITH THEIR CHARACTERISTIC FEATURES IN PARENTHESES

- *Portal hypertension (Cirrhosis and NCPH)*
- *Malignancy*: Lymphoma (also, presence of fatigue, frequent infections, easy bruising, skin rashes, palpable lymph nodes and presence of constitutional B symptoms: Pel–Ebstein fever of Hodgkin's lymphoma, night sweats, unexplained weight loss), leukemia
- *Hereditary spherocytosis (anemia, jaundice, gallstones)*
- *Idiopathic thrombocytopenic purpura (easy bruising, bleeding from the gums, heavy menstrual bleeding, petechiae*: A skin rash that looks like pinpoint red spots, fatigue.
- *Acute ITP*: Children ages 2–6, and symptoms usually disappear within 6 months
- *Chronic ITP*: Lasts 6 months or longer and is most commonly seen in adults
- *Splenic cyst*: Parasitic cyst (hydatid cyst) (most common), pseudocyst, true cyst
- *Splenic abscess*
- *Infection*: Malaria, kala-azar, typhoid, CMV, EBV, TB
- *Tropical splenomegaly*: Hyper-reactive malarial splenomegaly (HMS) caused by an exaggerated immune response to repeated malaria infections.
- *Felty syndrome*: It is a rare, severe form of RA that is also known as "super rheumatoid" disease. The triad of three conditions: Rheumatoid arthritis (RA), neutropenia, and splenomegaly.
- *Sarcoidosis*
- *Storage disorders (Gaucher and Niemann–Pick disease)*

ADRENAL MASS: Adenoma, Pheochromocytoma

RENAL MASS

OMENTAL LESION: Cyst, Metastasis, Tuberculous Involvement

RETROPERITONEAL MASS: PALN Mass/Lymphoma

■ REFERENCES

1. Agudelo Higuita NI, Brunetti E, McCloskey C. Cystic echinococcosis. Journal of clinical microbiology. 2016;54(3):518-23.
2. Anand S, Rajagopalan S, Mohan R. Management of liver hydatid cysts–Current perspectives. Medical journal armed forces India. 2012;68(3):304-9.
3. Schnelldorfer T, Torres VE, Zakaria S, Rosen CB, Nagorney DM. Polycystic liver disease: a critical appraisal of hepatic resection, cyst fenestration, and liver transplantation. Annals of surgery. 2009;250(1):112-8.

CHAPTER 9

Electrolytes and Calories in Two Minutes

ELECTROLYTES IN BODILY FLUIDS

- *Stomach*: Remember stomach is full of HCl (H$^+$ ions and highest Cl 130 mEq/L), so replacement best with isolyte G
- *Pancreatobiliary secretions*: High Na 145 mEq/L and Cl ~100 mEq/L, but potassium ~5 mEq/L
- *Pancreatic*: Highest bicarbonate (115 mEq/L)
- Same juices go into duodenum and ileum, so they have similar composition, except bicarbonate is ~30 mEq/L
- *Colon*: Highest potassium (30 mEq/L)

How to Treat Dyselectrolytemia

- *Hyponatremia*: Hypertonic saline 3% given at 1–2 mL/kg/h, the rate of sodium correction should be 6–12 mEq/L in the first 24 hours and 18 mEq/L or less in 48 hours. A bolus of 100–150 mL of hypertonic 3% saline can be given to correct severe hyponatremia.
- *Hypernatremia*: Half normal saline (0.45% NS), made in D5
- *Hypokalemia*: 2.5–3.5 mEq/L (representing mild-to-moderate hypokalemia), may need only oral potassium replacement.
  - If potassium levels are less than 2.5 mEq/L, intravenous (IV) potassium should be given.
  - Every 10 mEq of potassium increases serum potassium by 0.13 mEq/L. [Give (body weight × deficit) ÷ 3 along with daily requirements].
  - 20–40 mmoL potassium chloride in 1 L of sodium chloride 0.9% over at least 8 hours into a large vein.
- *Hyperkalemia*: Calcium gluconate or insulin + glucose.

Fluids

Post 28 days of life, isotonic fluids only shsould be used for resuscitation and maintenance.

Hypotonic fluids like half normal DNS, isolyte P, etc., should be used only in the first 28 days of life.

HOW TO CALCULATE CALORIC REQUIREMENT

Remember that:

$$\text{Total Energy Expenditure (TEE)} = \text{REE} \times \text{Activity factor (A)} \times \text{Stress factor (S)} \times \text{Fever (F)}$$

where A is 1.1 for ventilator dependent, 1.2 is bed ridden, 1.3 is mobilized, S is as per minor/major surgery, sepsis, etc., and F is 1 + 0.09 for every 0.5° rise above 38.5°C.

- Calculate basal metabolic rate (BMR)/REE (resting energy expenditure) as per Harris–Benedict equation (depends on age, height, weight)
- Multiply by A [1.1/1.2/1.3] and S [1.5/1.6 cancer cachexia/sepsis (major surgery)] and F [1 + 0.09 for every 0.5° rise above 38.5°C]
- That gives TEE which gives the total energy requirement
- Now, e.g., general energy requirement for 70 kg person is 25–35 kcal/kg/day (changes as per points 1–3), (ideally to be calculated as described above)
- Of that, protein intake must be 0.8 g/kg/day for normal, 1.5–2 g for hospitalized/major surgery and up to 3 g for severe sepsis (add 15–30 g more for per litre of fluid from an open abdomen)
- Of total energy, 20% must be from lipid
- Remaining are from carbs
- *1 g of carbs*: 3.4 kcal, 1 g protein: 4 kcal, 1 g lipid: 9 kcal, accordingly, total grams/calories distributed and calculated in diet.

10 CHAPTER

TNM Staging of Gastrointestinal and Hepatopancreatobiliary Cancers

TABLE 1: Esophagus	
Category	Criteria
T category	
TX	Tumor cannot be assessed
T0	No evidence of primary tumor
Tis	High-grade dysplasia, defined as malignant cells confined by the basement membrane
T1	Tumor invades the lamina propria, muscularis mucosae, or submucosa
T1a*	Tumor invades the lamina propria or muscularis mucosae
T1b*	Tumor invades the submucosa
T2	Tumor invades the muscularis propria
T3	Tumor invades the adventitia
T4	Tumor invades adjacent structures
T4a*	Tumor invades the pleura, pericardium, azygos vein, diaphragm, or peritoneum
T4b*	Tumor invades other adjacent structures, such as the aorta, vertebral body, or trachea
N category	
NX	Regional lymph nodes cannot be assessed
N0	No regional lymph node metastasis
N1	Metastasis in 1–2 regional lymph nodes
N2	Metastasis in 3–6 regional lymph nodes
N3	Metastasis in 7 or more regional lymph nodes
M category	
M0	No distant metastasis
M1	Distant metastasis

Continued

Continued

Category	Criteria
Adenocarcinoma G category	
GX	Differentiation cannot be assessed
G1	*Well-differentiated*: >95% of tumor is composed of well-formed glands
G2	*Moderately differentiated*: 50–95% of tumor shows gland formation
G3†	*Poorly differentiated*: Tumors composed of nest and sheets of cells with <50% of tumor demonstrating glandular formation
Squamous cell carcinoma G category	
GX	Differentiation cannot be assessed
G1	*Well-differentiated*: Prominent keratinization with pearl formation and a minor component of non-keratinizing basal-like cells. Tumor cells are arranged in sheets, and mitotic counts are low
G2	*Moderately differentiated*: Variable histologic features, ranging from parakeratotic to poorly keratinizing lesions. Generally, pearl formation is absent
G3‡	*Poorly differentiated*: Consists predominantly of basal-like cells forming large and small nests with frequent central necrosis. The nests consist of sheets or pavement-like arrangements of tumor cells, occasionally punctuated by small numbers of parakeratotic or keratinizing cells
*Squamous cell carcinoma L category***	
LX	Location unknown
Upper	Cervical esophagus to lower border of azygos vein
Middle	Lower border of azygos vein to lower border of inferior pulmonary vein
Lower	Lower border of inferior pulmonary vein to stomach, including esophagogastric junction

*Subcategories.
†If further testing of "undifferentiated" cancers reveals a glandular component, categorize as adenocarcinoma G3.
‡If further testing of "undifferentiated" cancers reveals a squamous cell component, or if after further testing they remain undifferentiated, categorize as squamous cell carcinoma G3.
**Location is defined by the epicentre of the esophageal tumor.

TABLE 2: Stomach

Category	Criteria
T category	
TX	Primary tumor cannot be assessed
T0	No evidence of primary tumor
Tis	*Carcinoma in situ*: Intraepithelial tumor without invasion of the lamina propria, high-grade dysplasia
T1	Tumor invades the lamina propria, muscularis mucosae, or submucosa
T1a	Tumor invades the lamina propria or muscularis mucosae
T1b	Tumor invades the submucosa
T2	Tumor invades the muscularis propria

Continued

Continued

Category	Criteria
T3	Tumor invades the subserosal connective tissue without invasion of the visceral peritoneum or adjacent structures
T4	Tumor invades the serosa (visceral peritoneum) or adjacent structures
T4a	Tumor invades the serosa (visceral peritoneum)
T4b	Tumor invades adjacent structures/organs
N category	
NX	Regional lymph nodes cannot be assessed
N0	No regional lymph node metastasis
N1	Metastases in 1–2 regional lymph nodes
N2	Metastases in 3–6 regional lymph nodes
N3	Metastases in ≥7 regional lymph nodes
N3a	Metastases in 7 or 15 regional lymph nodes
N3b	Metastases in 16 or more regional lymph nodes
M category	
M0	No distant metastasis
M1	Distant metastasis

(AJCC: American Joint Committee on Cancer; UICC: Union for International Cancer Control)
Source: Stomach Cancer TNM Staging AJCC UICC 8th Edition.

TABLE 3A: American Joint Committee on Cancer (AJCC) TNM staging classification for colorectal cancer 8th ed., 2017

T	Primary tumor
Tx	Primary tumor cannot be assessed
T0	No evidence of primary tumor
Tis	Carcinoma in situ (invasion of lamina propria)
T1	Tumor invades submucosa
T2	Tumor invades muscularis propria
T3	Tumor invades subserosa or into non-peritonealized pericolic or perirectal tissue
T4	Tumor directly invades other organs or structures and/or perforates visceral peritoneum
T4a	Tumor perforates visceral peritoneum
T4b	Tumor directly invades other organs or structures

Continued

Continued

N	Regional nodes
Nx	Regional nodes cannot be assessed
N0	No regional lymph nodes identified

N	Regional nodes
N1	Metastasis in one to three lymph nodes (tumor in lymph nodes measuring ≥0.2 mm) or any number of tumor deposits are present, and all identifiable lymph nodes are negative
N1a	Metastasis in one regional lymph node
N1b	Metastasis in two to three regional lymph nodes
N1c	No regional lymph nodes are positive, but there are tumor deposits (i.e., satellites in the subserosa or in non-peritonealized pericolic or perirectal soft tissue) without lymph node metastasis
N2	Metastasis in four or more regional lymph nodes
N2a	Metastasis in four to six regional lymph nodes
N2b	Metastasis in seven or more regional lymph nodes

M	Distant metastasis
M0	No distant metastasis
M1	Distant metastasis
M1a	Metastasis confined to one organ (liver, lung, ovary, non-regional lymph nodes) without peritoneal metastasis
M1b	Metastasis to more than one organ
M1c	Metastasis to the peritoneum with or without other organ involvement

T categories: Although these categories have not changed and T4 was divided into T4a and T4b in the previous edition, further clarification was made that tumors with perforation in which tumor cells are continuous with the serosal surface through an inflammatory reaction are considered at least T4a. In the absence of proven perforation, tumors that invade only adjacent organs or structures are considered T4b.

N categories: There is discussion regarding isolated tumor cells in lymph nodes and micrometastases. Isolated tumor cells consist of up to 20 cells within lymph node sinuses or the medullary sinus of lymph nodes. These should be designated as N0 (i.e., N0i+), but their presence does not change the N category.

Micrometastases are clusters of 20 or more cells or metastases measuring >0.2 mm and <2 mm in diameter. Lymph nodes with micrometastases are considered positive and designated N1.

The interpretation of tumor deposits remains the same. Nodes that contain no identifiable lymphoid tissue or show angiolymphatic invasion should be considered tumor deposits and designated as N1c. Tumor deposits within areas of the visceral wall should be considered lymphovascular invasion with site-specific designations of L+ (for lymphatic invasion) and V+ (for deposits in endothelial cell-lined spaces with associated thrombus). If tumor nodules are found in the peritoneal surface, they are classified as peritoneal carcinomatosis under M1c.

The number of tumor deposits does not influence the N category and is not added to the number of positive nodes.

M categories: M1c, which denotes peritoneal metastases, has been added.

TABLE 3B: Colorectal Stage Grouping

0	Tis	N0	M0
I	T1–T2		
IIA	T3		
IIB	T4a		
IIC	T4b		
IIIA	• T1–T2 • T1	• N1/N1c • N2a	
IIIB	• T3–T4a • T2–T3 • T1–T2	• N1/N1c • N2a • N2b	
IIIC	• T4a • T3–T4a • T4b	• N2a • N2b • N1–N2	
IVA	Any T	Any N	M1a
IVB			M1b
IVC			M1c

TABLE 4: Gallbladder cancer (GBC)

T	T criteria
TX	Primary tumor cannot be assessed
T0	No evidence of primary tumor
Tis	Carcinoma in situ
T1	Tumor invades the lamina propria or muscular layer
T1a	Tumor invades the lamina propria
T1b	Tumor invades the muscular layer
T2	Tumor invades the perimuscular connective tissue on the peritoneal side, without involvement of the serosa (visceral peritoneum) or tumor invades the perimuscular connective tissue on the hepatic side, with no extension into the liver
T2a	Tumor invades the perimuscular connective tissue on the peritoneal side, without involvement of the serosa (visceral peritoneum)
T2b	Tumor invades the perimuscular connective tissue on the hepatic side, with no extension into the liver
T3	Tumor perforates the serosa (visceral peritoneum) and/or directly invades the liver and/or one other adjacent organ or structure, such as the stomach, duodenum, colon, pancreas, omentum, or extrahepatic bile ducts
T4	Tumor invades the main portal vein or hepatic artery or invades two or more extrahepatic organs or structures

Continued

Continued

N	N criteria (at least ≥ 6 LNs)
NX	Regional LN cannot be assessed
N0	No regional LN metastasis
N1	Metastases to 1–3 regional LNs
N2	Metastases to ≥ 4 regional LNs
M	**M criteria**
M0	No distant metastasis
M1	Distant metastasis present

T	N	M	Stage
Tis	N0	M0	0
T1	N0	M0	I
T2a	N0	M0	IIA
T2b	N0	M0	IIB
T3	N0	M0	IIIA
T1–3	N1	M0	IIIB
T4	N0–1	M0	IIIB
Any T	N2	M0	IVB
Any T	Any N	M1	IVB

TABLE 5: Hepatocellular carcinoma (HCC)						
	Primary tumor (T)		**Regional lymph nodes (N)**		**Distant metastases (M)**	
T1a	Solitary tumor ≤2 cm with/without vascular invasion	Nx	Regional lymph nodes cannot be assessed	M0	No distant metastasis
T1b	Solitary tumor >2 cm without vascular invasion	N0	No regional lymph node metastasis	M1	Distant metastasis
T2	Solitary tumor >2 cm with vascular invasion or multifocal tumors, none >5 cm	N1	Regional lymph node metastasis		
T3	Multifocal tumors at least one of which is >5 cm				
T4	Single tumor or multifocal tumors of any size involving a major branch of the portal vein or hepatic vein or tumor(s) with direct invasion of adjacent organs other than the gallbladder or with perforation of visceral peritoneum				

Continued

Continued

Stage classification			
Stage	T	N	M
IA	T1a	N0	M0
IB	T1b	N0	M0
II	T2	N0	M0
IIIA	T3	N0	M0
IIIB	T4	N0	M0
IVA	Any T	N1	M0
IVB	Any T	Any N	M1

Source: AJCC 8th Edition Staging System for Hepatocellular Carcinoma.

TABLE 6: Intrahepatic cholangiocarcinoma (IHCC)

8th edition AJCC

T1a	Solitary tumor ≤5 cm without vascular invasion
T1b	Solitary tumor >5 cm without vascular invasion
T2	Solitary tumor with intrahepatic vascular invasion or multiple tumors, with or without vascular invasion
T3	Tumor perforating the visceral peritoneum
T4	Tumor involving local extrahepatic structures by direct invasion

8th edition AJCC

N0	No regional lymph node metastasis		
N1	Regional lymph node metastasis present		
IA	T1a	N0	M0
IB	T1b	N0	M0
II	T2	N0	M0
IIIA	T3	N0	M0
IIIB	T4	N1	M0
IV	Any T	Any N	M1

TABLE 7: Perihilar cholangiocarcinoma (pHCC)

8th edition AJCC

T category (pT)

Tis	Carcinoma in situ/high-grade dysplasia
T1	Confined to the bile duct, with extension up to the muscle layer or fibrous tissue
T2	Invades beyond the wall of the bile duct, or adjacent hepatic parenchyma
T2a	Invades beyond the wall of the bile duct to surrounding adipose tissue
T2b	Invades adjacent hepatic parenchyma

Continued

Continued

8th edition AJCC

T category (pT)

T3	Invades unilateral branches of the portal vein or hepatic artery
T4	Invades the main portal vein or its branches bilaterally, or the common hepatic artery; or unilateral second-order biliary radicals with contralateral portal vein or hepatic artery involvement

N category (pN)

N0	No regional lymph node metastasis
N1	Metastasis to 1–3 regional lymph nodes
N2	Metastasis to ≥4 regional lymph nodes

AJCC stage groupings	T	N	M
I	T1	N0	M0
II	T2a–b	N0	M0
IIIA	T3	N0	M0
IIIB	T4	N0	M0
IIIC	Any T	N1	M0
IVA	Any T	N2	M0
IVB	Any T	Any N	M1

TABLE 8: Distal extrahepatic bile duct (EHBD)

8th edition AJCC

T category (pT)

Tis	Carcinoma in situ/high-grade dysplasia
T1	Invades the bile duct wall with a depth <5 mm
T2	Invades the bile duct wall with a depth of 5–12 mm
T3	Invades the bile duct wall with a depth >12 mm
T4	Involves the celiac axis, superior mesenteric artery, and/or common hepatic artery

N category (pN)

N0	No regional lymph node metastasis
N1	Metastasis in 1–3 regional lymph nodes
N2	Metastasis in ≥4 regional lymph nodes

AJCC stage groupings	T	N	M
I	T1	N0	M0
IA	–	–	–
IB	–	–	–
IIA	• T1 • T2	• N1 • N0	• M0 • M0
IIB	• T2 • T3	• N1 • N0–1	• M0 • M0

Continued

CHAPTER 10: TNM Staging of Gastrointestinal and Hepatopancreatobiliary Cancers

Continued

AJCC stage groupings	T	N	M
IIIA	T1–3	N2	M0
IIIB	T4	Any N	M0
III	–	–	–
IV	Any T	Any N	M1

TABLE 9: Pancreas	
8th edition: Exocrine pancreas	**8th edition: Endocrine pancreas**
T category (pT)	
Tis	Carcinoma in situ	Limited to the pancreas, <2 cm
T1	≤2 cm	
T1a	≤0.5 cm	
T1b	>0.5 cm and <1 cm	
T1c	1–2 cm	
T2	>2 cm and ≤4 cm	Limited to the pancreas, 2–4 cm
T3	>4 cm	Limited to the pancreas, >4 cm; or invading the duodenum or common bile duct
T4	Involves the celiac axis, superior mesenteric artery, and/or common hepatic artery	Invading adjacent organs or the wall of large vessels
8th edition: Exocrine pancreas	**8th edition: Endocrine pancreas**
N category (pN)	
N0	No regional lymph node metastasis	No regional lymph node involvement
N1	Metastasis in 1–3 regional lymph nodes	Regional lymph node involvement
N2	Metastasis in ≥4 regional lymph nodes	
AJCC stage groupings	
IA	T1 N0 M0	T1 N0 M0
IB	T2 N0 M0	
I		T1 N0 M0
IIA	T3 N0 M0	
IIB	T1–3 N1 M0	
II		T2–3 N0 M0
III	T1–3 N2 M0; T4 any N M0	T4 N0 M0; any T N1 M0
IV	Any T any N M1	Any T any N M1

11 Clinical Trials

■ ESOPHAGUS AND GASTROESOPHAGEAL JUNCTION (GEJ) CANCER

French FFCD: Perioperative 3# CF better OS.
MAGIC: 3# ECF before and after surgery. Better OS.
FLOT4: 4# FLOT before and after surgery. Better OS.

NeoFLOT for GEJ adenocarcinoma: 6#FLOT as intensive NACT doesn't increase preoperative complications, but had increased blood transfusion requirements.

FLOT is preferred for poorly differentiated tumors (as they are less responsive to ECF), but at the expense of increased toxicity (cytopenias, neuro, hepatic, renal toxicity, alopecia, mucositis, nausea, vomiting, diarrhea)

CROSS: NACRT (carboplatin + paclitaxel with 41.4 Grays), 1.8 Gy/day, 23# over 5 weeks, and surgery is done 6–8 weeks later. Pathological complete response (pCR): 49% for SCC and 23% for adenoCA.

PROTECT: CROSS versus 3#FOLFOX-RT (41.4 Gy) for esophageal and junctional cancer.

Results: Both provided short-term benefit on R0 resection; however, CP is associated with a severe postoperative morbidity rate higher than expected.

NEOSCOPE: Compared induction chemo with CAPOX followed by either CAPOX-RT or carboplatin/paclitaxel-RT (45 Gy).

So long-term evidence showed that induction CAPOX followed by switch to CarPac-RT was superior to CAPOX-RT, with similar efficacy as seen in CROSS and FLOT.

TOP GEAR trial for GEJ adenocarcinoma with perioperative ECF chemo versus perioperative chemoRT (2#ECF followed by 5-FU based RT followed by surgery and adjuvant 3#ECF showed that addition of RT is safe without additional morbidity).

Neo-AEGIS trial (only adenocarcinoma histology) [178 CROSS, 184 MAGIC/FLOT (157/27)]

So perioperative chemo is NOT inferior to CROSS.

Also, chemo arm of MAGIC (83%), no longer represents the standard after the publication of FLOT data. According to histopathological regression analysis of the FLOT trial, the pCR rate of the FLOT arm is 16%, which was only 5% in the EOX arm of the Neo-AEGIS trial.

ESOPEC trial: CROSS versus FLOT, so FLOT has better pCR and OS and is now the SOC for resectable EAC.

MUNICON 1 trial (Siewert 1 and 2 adenoca, T3, T4, N+): PET/CT done at baseline.

NACT: CF and folinic acid +– paclitaxel for good PS.

Assessed with FDG PET CT after 2 weeks of starting NACT. So responders defined as those having ≥35% reduction in SUV_{max}. Responders have better prognosis and are given complete course of NACT (over 12 weeks) followed 4–6 weeks later by surgery, as compared with non-responders, who are taken for surgery directly after 2 weeks of NACT (lesser PFS, OS than responders, but better than non-responders who keep continuing ineffective chemo).

MUNICON 2 trial: Non-responders given salvage chemoradiotherapy (cisplatin or 5-FU based 32 Gy RT) for 12 weeks, followed by surgery. However, their prognosis was still poor (better HPE response, but no improvement in R0 resection rate) as compared with responders, which showed that poor biology disease has a poor prognosis.

Next Trial (JCOG) for esophageal SCC: Neoadjuvant CF (cisplatin 80 mg/m² on day 1 plus 5-FU 800 mg/m² on days 1–5 Q3W/2 course), DCF (docetaxel 70 mg/m² on day 1, cisplatin 70 mg/m² on day 1, plus 5-FU 750 mg/m² on days 1–5 Q3W/3 course), or CF-RT.

The 3-year PFS was 47.7%, 61.8%, and 58.5%, respectively. R0 resection was achieved in 168 (84.4%), 173 (85.6%), and 175 (87.5%), and pCR was 4 (2.1%), 40 (19.8%), and 77 (38.5%), respectively.

Conclusion: DCF significantly improved PFS and OS over CF as neoadjuvant therapy for locally advanced ESCC, with a manageable toxicity profile. DCF represents a new standard neoadjuvant treatment for ESCC.

TIGER study: Distribution of LN metastases in esophageal CA.

SNAP study: Role of sentinel node (SN) surgery after endoscopic radical resection in CA esophagus.

Watch-and-wait (WW) trials in esophageal CA: ESOSTRATE, ESOPRESSO, PRIDE, SANO.

PREPARE study: Role of preoperative incentive spirometry in reducing postoperative pneumonia.

NUTRIENT 2 trial: Early versus delayed start of orals after MIE/Hybrid Surgery.

Robot assisted minimally invasive esophagectomy (RAMIE): There is evidence that patients with cT4b tumors can be safely treated with RAMIE after LC-CRT and restaging with PET-CT.

ROBOT trial: RAMIE versus open transthoracic esophagectomy (TTE). So RAMIE can achieve shorter operative duration and better lymph node dissection in patients who received neoadjuvant therapy.

■ GEJ/GASTRIC CANCER

ACTS GC: Role of adjuvant S1 in GC.
CLASSIC, ARTIST: For adjuvant chemo
CLASSIC trial in GC: Adjuvant CAPOX has better OS than surgery only (D2)

ARTIST 1 *for resected D2 GC*: XP versus XP+XRT+XP. The addition of XRT to XP chemotherapy did not significantly prolong DFS. However, in the subgroup of patients with pathologic lymph node metastasis at the time of surgery, patients randomly assigned to the XP/XRT/XP arm experienced superior DFS when compared with those who received XP alone.

ARTIST 2 *for resected D2 node + stage 2/3 GC*: Adjuvant S1 versus SOX versus SOXRT. So adjuvant SOX and SOXRT are better than S1 monotherapy and improve DFS. However, addition of RT to SOX does not improve rate of recurrence.

CRITICS *trial in GC*: Adjuvant CRT did not improve OS, as compared to adequate preoperative chemo with D2 resection.

FLOT3 for oligometastatic disease (OS 31 months for NACT of 4# FLOT followed by curative resection of primary and metastases, followed by adjuvant chemo of 4# FLOT vs. 16 months only for 8# FLOT followed by noncurative resection)

FLOT4: FLOT is superior to ECF. Almost 37% major HPE response which was close to the CRT protocols, which formed the basis for the ESOPEC study. (ESOPEC later proved FLOT to be better than CROSS).

ONGOING FLOT 5 RENAISSANCE trial and SURGIGAST trial for oligometastatic GEJ/GC

DANTE FLOT 8: Perioperative FLOT + Atezolizumab versus Only Perioperative FLOT for GEJ CA and LAGC.

FLOT 9: Prophylactic HIPEC in signet ring CA as it has high risk for metastases (NACT FLOT followed by surgery with HIPEC followed by adjuvant FLOT)

CYTO-CHIP *study for peritoneal metastases positive GC*: CRS-HIPEC improves OS compared with cytoreductive surgery (CRS) alone.

GASTRIPEC *study for peritoneal metastases positive GC*: CRS+HIPEC versus CRS alone.

So HIPEC did not add to OS, but improved PFS and other metastasis free survival, as problem with study was that almost 50% had peritoneal carcinomatosis index score (PCI) >7 with ascites which are poor prognostic factors. However, subgroup analysis showed that for patients undergoing complete cytoreduction, there was definite increase in OS in CRS + HIPEC group compared with CRS alone.

CARDIA trial for transthoracic esophagectomy (TTE) versus transhiatal extended gastrectomy (THEG) for Siewert 2 (adenoCA obviously) is going on.

Siewert classification is only 50–60% accurate for exact location (EUS, CT). Frozen section for proximal margin after THEG, has false negatives in poorly differentiated, submucosal spread, after NAT and due to stapler artefact.

Targeted Therapy

Trastuzumab in HER2+ for perioperative/NACT/metastatic GEJ/gastric cancer (GC):
- ***RTOG*** (esophageal CA) and ***TOGA*** (XP+Trastuzumab in GC)
- ***PETRARCA*** for pertuzumab with perioperative FLOT.
- ***INNOVATION*** and ***TRAP*** for both.

In HER2-negative GEJ and gastric adenoca:
RAMSES, REGARD, RAINBOW for VEGFR-2 antibody ramucirumab with perioperative FLOT.

Also, ***GLOW*** and ***SPOTLIGHT*** trials for Zolbetuximab, which is the newest drug and will be a first-line treatment option for CLDN18.2+, HER2-negative, advanced unresectable metastatic GC/GEJ CA.

PD-L1 inhibitors (for MMR deficient/MSI high tumors):
Keynote-811 is a phase III trial where patients with HER2-positive metastatic gastric or GEJC were randomized either to pembrolizumab + standard of care (SOC being anti-HER2 and chemotherapy) or placebo + SOC. Adding pembrolizumab to SOC resulted in a substantial, statistically significant increase in ORR as first-line therapy for HER2+ metastatic G/GEJ cancer.

CheckMate 649 trial:
Nivolumab (anti PD-L1) + chemo became standard in advanced or metastatic EC/GEJ and GC.

Moonlight trial:
Role of PD L1 inhibitor in metastatic GC. FOLFOX versus FOLFOX + Nivolumab and Ipilimumab.

Perfect:
Addition of Atezolizumab to CROSS.

■ COLORECTAL

Colon Cancer

Neoadjuvant chemotherapy:
FOxTROT trial (NACT for locally advanced colon cancer: T3/4 or N+ vs. upfront surgery 6 weeks of NACT given).

So FOLFOX based NACT led to significant tumor downstaging, fewer positive margins and fewer apical LN involvement, and thus reduced the 2-year recurrence rate.

Even NCCN recommends NACT for T4b cancers, as there are reports showing that it also improves OS, while NACRT can be given for colon cancers infiltrating duodenum/pancreas and sigmoid cancers infiltrating bladder/vagina, provided small bowel can be safeguarded.

Adjuvant chemotherapy:
- NSABP (5-FU and Leucovorin based)
- MOSAIC (established FOLFOX for stage 3)

IDEA trial: 13,000 stage 3 randomized to 3 or 6 months of adjuvant CAPOX or FOLFOX. For low-risk stage 3 (T1-3/N1), 3 months CAPOX is non-inferior to 6. But 3 months FOLFOX is inferior to 6. Whereas for high-risk stage 3 (T4/N2), 3 months of both CAPOX or FOLFOX are inferior to 6. Based on this, NCCN recommends 3 months CAPOX OR 6 months FOLFOX for low-risk stage 3, but 6 months CAPOX OR FOLFOX for high-risk stage 3.

NSABP, MOSAIC, ASCO: For high-risk stage 2 (T4, obstructed, perforated, <12 LN harvested, poorly differentiated, close margins, tumor budding/LVI/PNI+): Capecitabine or 5-FU/Leucovorin adjuvant chemo must be given. Oxaliplatin must be added if tumor is MMR deficient as it won't respond to 5-FU alone.

Rectal Cancer

Neoadjuvant chemotherapy (NACT) alone:
- **PROSPECT** (FOLFOX with selective LC-CRT for those not responding)
- **BACCHUS** (FOLFOX vs. FOLFOXIRI, both with bevacizumab, total 6 cycles)

Radiotherapy (RT) alone
Stockholm-3:
- Short course radiotherapy (SCRT) with immediate surgery versus
- SCRT with delayed surgery (4–8 weeks) versus
- Long-course radiotherapy (LCRT) with delayed surgery (4–8 weeks)
- So SCRT with delayed surgery safe with highest pCR among the 3

TRIMODAL regimen (NACRT-surgery-chemo)
NCCN 2020 guidelines: Total 6 months of preoperative therapy [total neoadjuvant therapy (TNT) or usual trimodal regimen].

For stage II/III mid and low rectal cancer, SCRT (not for T4 if given solo, i.e., if not part of TNT) or LC-CRT followed by surgery, and systemic chemo given either before (becomes TNT) or after surgery (usual trimodal regimen).

They recommend adjuvant chemo for clinical stage II/III rectal cancer who received neoadjuvant radiation, regardless of final histology.

Now for deciding SCRT versus LC-CRT as part of *usual trimodal regimen*
LC-CRT preferred for T4/threatened or positive CRM, as it sterilizes, downstages and increases chance of organ preservation, whereas SCRT only sterilizes. However, SCRT *when used as part of TNT*, is a valid treatment option for all advanced tumors (T3/4, N+, EMVI+, CRM+, pelvic sidewall N+) and has been used in all consolidation versus standard trials.

Adjuvant therapy when NAC/CRT not given (Tumor mis-staged by MRI ~25–30%), NCCN 2020 guidelines:
- Total 6 months of therapy.
- For low-risk stage II (pT3, negative CRM), adjuvant chemoRT followed by capecitabine OR 5-FU/leucovorin is preferred, but observation alone is also an option.
- For high-risk stage II (pT4, positive CRM, positive margins) or any stage III, adjuvant chemoRT followed by CAPOX or FOLFOX is preferred.

However, many argue that benefit of postoperative RT may be minimal if negative CRM and margins are achieved as compared to it is toxicity, and that current chemo regimens are highly effective. Thus, another reasonable strategy is to treat N+ but negative CRM and margins, with postoperative chemo only.

Total neoadjuvant therapy trials:
- *TNT advantages*: Higher compliance and systemic chemo completion, higher clinical complete response (cCR) enabling WW for organ preservation, higher pCR (almost double) and pCR in consolidation greater than induction, lower margin positivity, lower loco regional recurrence, lower distant metastases rate, and thus better DFS with TNT.
- TNT is generally followed by surgery.
- Now if with advanced tumors/high-risk features (indication for preoperative chemoRT), cCR is seen, then there is an option of WW, which becomes accidental WW.
- But if the patient desires organ preservation for mid/low rectal tumors, then even if there is no indication for preoperative chemoRT (i.e., early tumors/no high-risk features), intentional WW with a view to organ preservation can be done using TNT.

Induction chemo trials (NACT followed by chemoRT): Mnemonic ACE
- **AVACROSS**
- **CONTRE 2**
- **COPERNICUS (UK)**
- **EXPERT**
- **EXPERT C**

Consolidation chemo landmark trial:
Angelita Habr-Gama's refined TNT protocol for T3/4 and/or N+ rectal cancers: Infusional 5-FU and Leucovorin 3 cycles-based 45 Grays RT over 5 weeks with 9 Grays boost followed by 3 cycles of infusional 5-FU/Leucovorin, followed by tumor assessment after 8 weeks, with latest report showing cCR of 68%, with 5-year DFS of 60%.

Induction versus standard:
- **PRODIGE** (6# FOLFIRINOX followed by chemoRT)

Consolidation versus standard (all used SCRT):
- **RAPIDO:** CAPEOX/FOLFOX used
- **POLISH 2:** Only 3# CAPEOX
- **STELLAR:** 4#CAPEOX before surgery, and 2# after

Induction versus consolidation (all used LC-CRT):
- **AIO/ARO/CAO**
- **OPRA**
- **COLOR 3 (ongoing):** TaTME versus Lap TME.

Ileocecal crohn's
- **LIRIC trial** (lap ileocecal resection vs. infliximab in terminal ileitis of crohn's) showed that laparoscopic ileocaecal resection is a better treatment option than infliximab, in patients with Crohn's disease with limited (affected segment ≤40 cm) and predominantly inflammatory terminal ileitis for whom conventional treatment (non-biological) is not successful. So 5 years later, none of the resection patients required a re-resection and only 25% required biological, whereas in those who were in the infliximab arm, 50% needed surgery and the other 50% were still on infliximab. Thus, for ileocecal Crohn's, upfront resection can be preferred over medical treatment.

For Perianal Fistulas in Crohn's
PISA trial: So Seton versus infliximab versus Surgical closure + Infliximab for high fistulas. Outcome: Surgical closure + Infliximab had better closure rates. Hence early surgery recommended.

Rectal prolapse
PROSPER trial: Equal recurrence rates between peroneal and abdominal rectopexy procedures.

Criteria for CRS in GI Cancers
- *Colorectal cancer*: PCI ≤15
- *Gastric cancer*: PCI ≤ 6 and HIPEC needs complete/near complete cytoreduction (CC0/CC1, so largest nodule is <2.5 mm as beyond that, drug penetration is poor)

PIPAC (Oxaliplatin or cisplatin-doxorubicin) is given mostly in palliative setting, alternating 6 weekly (+–2 weeks) with systemic chemo (FLOT, ECF, EOX, FOLFIRI), but can also be given as NACT for unresectable peritoneal metastases which can be followed up with secondary CRS and HIPEC if PCI scores fall into resectable category, without any ascites, followed by adjuvant chemo.

■ PANCREAS

Pancreatic Cancer
Three preoperative scores that predict poor prognosis as per ISGPS 2014 paper on borderline resectable pancreatic cancer:
1. Modified Glasgow Prognostic Score (mGPS 0, 1, 2) based on CRP (<10 to >10) and albumin (<3.5 in score 2)
   So mGPS 0: Best OS, and mGPS 2 worst OS
2. Neutrophil/lymphocytes ratio >5 = Poor OS, and superior score to mGPS
3. CA 19-9 ≥1,000 has resection rate of only 15.4% and ≥4,000, 5-year survival is 0%.

Also, BRPC A, B, C given first by MD Anderson group, followed by IAP consensus definitions in Sendai, Japan, in 2016.

NACT:
- **PREOPANC 1:** Neoadjuvant gemcitabine-based CRT followed by surgery and adjuvant GEM improves OS compared with upfront surgery and adjuvant gemcitabine in resectable and BRPC.
- **PREOPANC 2:** TNT with FOLFIRINOX did not improve OS as compared with GEM-based CRT followed by surgery and adjuvant GEM.
- **ESPAC 5 (previously 5f):** Compared short course NATs (GEMCAP inspired from ESPAC 4, vs. FOLFIRINOX inspired from PRODIGE, vs. CAP-CRT) versus upfront surgery.
  - So short course (8 weeks) NAT has similar resection rates, but better OS than upfront surgery in BRPC. NAT with either GEMCAP or FOLFIRINOX had better survival than with immediate surgery.
- **LATEST ALLIANCE trial** *A021501*: NACT mFOLFIRINOX alone was associated with favorable OS in BRPC compared with induction therapy with mFOLFIRINOX plus hypofractionated RT.

Adjuvant chemo trials for BRPC, after NACT already given:
AGEOFRENCH: Out of 80 who underwent surgery for BRPC after NACT FOLFIRINOX, only 54% of received adjuvant chemo; No improved survival.

NACT trials for purely resectable PDAC:
- **PREOPANC 3** (ongoing)
  Perioperative mFOLFIRINOX
- **NORPACT 1**- NO survival benefit with FOLFIRINOX versus upfront surgery
- **NEPAFOX**-Perioperative FOLFIRINOX versus Adjuvant GEM
  Shorter median survival with FFX seen.

Adjuvant:
- **CONKO-001**
  GEM versus observation.
  Statistically significant difference in survival with GEM (median OS 22.8 vs. 20.2 months, respectively, median DFS 13.4 vs. 6.9 months)

ESPAC 1- *So 5-FU versus 5-FU CRT*:
- Increased OS with 5-FU, and became standard of care (SOC).

ESPAC 3:
- 5-FU versus GEM.
- No difference in OS, but improved toxicity with GEM, and GEM became SOC.

ESPAC 4: Improved OS with GEMCAP versus GEM alone. So GEMCAP better.

ESPAC 6: Will utilise a signature panel in resected tumor, to stratify into GEM or OX based regimens.

JASPAC 01:
- S1 versus GEM.
- S1 better.

PRODIGE-24:
- mFOLFIRINOX versus GEM.
- mFOLFIRINOX regimen showed a longer survival than GEM (median OS was 54.4 vs. 35.0 months, median DFS 21.6 vs. 12.8 months, respectively)

APACT:
- GnP versus GEM alone.
- GnP didn't show any survival advantage over GEM and hence, is not licensed for use in the adjuvant setting.

Metastatic PDAC:
- ***PRODIGE:*** FOLFIRINOX reported to have a 11 months median OS, versus 6.8 months in GEM, and a PFS 6.4 versus 3.3 months, respectively.
- ***MPACT:*** GnP versus GEM alone, showing a 8.7 versus 6.6 months OS, and GnP group was also associated with a improved 1- and 2-year survival, response rate and PFS.
- ***POLO:*** Efficacy of olaparib, a PARP inhibitor, as maintenance therapy in those with germline BRCA1/2 mutation (PFS 7.4 vs. 3.8 months in placebo)

Surgical trials:
Open distal pancreatectomy (ODP) versus Lap DP (LDP):
- **LEOPARD 1:** LDP reduces time to functional recovery compared with ODP. Although the overall rate of complications was not reduced, LDP was associated with less delayed gastric emptying and better QOL without increasing costs.

Open Whipple versus Lap:
- **LEOPARD 2:** Poor results with laparoscopic pancreaticoduodenectomy (LPD), trial stopped prematurely
- **PADULAP:** 1-day shorter hospital stay in the LPD group, with similar short-term morbidity and mortality rates.

Other surgery trials:
- **PASIREOTIDE** reduce POPF rates.
- **RECOPANC:** PJ versus PG.
  Similar rates of grades B/C POPF. More PPH with PG.
- ***PANasta:*** Cattell warren PJ (duct to mucosa) versus Blumgart PJ (duct to mucosa + jejunal overlap).
  No difference in POPF seen.

Neuroendocrine Neoplasms (NEN)

Neuroendocrine neoplasms trials:
- So NENs comprise of NETs and NECs.
- Well differentiated NENs are called NETs (Grades 1 to 3 based on mitotic index and Ki 67), whereas poorly differentiated NENs are called NECs (Grade 3 by default).

For pNET:
1. ***RADIANT 3:*** Everolimus 10 mg versus Placebo
2. Sunitinib 37.5 mg versus Placebo

3. In the **OCLURANDOM trial**, PFS was longer in patients receiving Lu 177-octreotate PRRT versus sunitinib.
4. **ECOG 2211:** CAPTEM versus Temozolomide (CAPTEM best)

For non-pNET:
1. **PROMID:** Octreotide LAR 30 mg 4 weeks
2. **CLARINET:** Lanreotide autogel 120 mg 4 weeks
3. **RADIANT 2:** Everolimus 10 mg + Octreotide LAR 30 mg versus Octreotide LAR 30 mg
4. **RADIANT 4:** Everolimus 10 mg versus Placebo
5. **NETTER 1** – (midgut neuroendocrine tumors): Lu 177 DOTATE PRRT + Octreotide 30 mg versus Octreotide 60 mg
   ^{177}Lu-Dotatate treatment did not significantly improve median overall survival versus high-dose long-acting octreotide. Despite final overall survival not reaching statistical significance, the 11.7 month difference in median overall survival with ^{177}Lu-Dotatate treatment versus high-dose long-acting octreotide alone might be considered clinically relevant.
6. **NETTER 2** – (Lu-Dotatate plus long-acting octreotide vs. high-dose long-acting octreotide for the treatment of newly diagnosed, advanced grade 2–3, well-differentiated, gastroenteropancreatic neuroendocrine tumors): First-line ^{177}Lu-Dotatate plus octreotide LAR significantly extended median progression-free survival (by 14 months) in patients with grade 2 or 3 advanced gastroenteropancreatic neuroendocrine tumours. ^{177}Lu-Dotatate should be considered a new standard of care in first-line therapy in this population.

TELESTAR trial: Telotristat, inhibitor of tryptophan hydroxylase, inhibiting conversion of tryptophan to serotonin, for treatment of refractory diarrhea of carcinoid syndrome despite SSAs.

NEN (NET and NEC) management strategy:
- *For localized and even metastatic NET (G1, 2, 3)*: Surgery is first line, including debulking/CRS for metastases.
- *For localized NEC*: Radical resection
- *But for metastatic NEC*: No resection, only platinum/Etoposide based chemo.

If progressive/metastases, then for G1, G2:
- SSAs and PRRT are first line (as they possess SSTR-2). If not responding, then Everolimus and Sunitinib for pNETs.

If progressive/for metastatic G3 NET and NEC:
- Only option is cytotoxic chemo.
- So CAPTEM is best for metastatic G3 pNET.
- And Carboplatin/Etoposide as first line and FOLFOX/FOLFOXIRI as second line for metastatic GEP NEC.

Remember:
- *In MEN-1 associated pNEN*:
    - Observe for lesions ≤ 2 cm.
    - Operate for >2 cm.

Whereas for VHL associated pNEN:
- Observe for lesions ≤1.5 cm.
- Operate for >3 cm, exon 3 mutation and doubling time <500 days. (VHL: All is 3. Three letter word, chromosome 3p, operate >3 cm and if exon 3 mutation)

ADVANCED HCC (FOR SYSTEMIC THERAPY)

SHARP: Sorafenib

Noninferiority trials to sorafenib:
- **REFLECT:** Lenvatinib (oral multikinase inhibitor targeting VEGFR 1–3 and FGFR 1–4) found non-inferior to Sorafenib.
- **RATIONALE-301:** Most recently, Tislelizumab (PD1-inhibitor), found non-inferior to sorafenib.

Superiority trials to sorafenib:
a. **IMBrave150:** Atezolizumab-bevacizumab (Combination of PD-L1 inhibitor and VEGF inhibitor) superior PFS and OS than Sorafenib. Untreated or incompletely treated esophageal or gastric varices were excluded as a precautionary measure for bevacizumab—related risks. But now it is found to be safe even in Child B.
b. **HIMALAYA:** STRIDE regimen (Durvalumab-tremelimumab) superior to Sorafenib.

GALLBLADDER CANCER (GBC)/CHOLANGIOCARCINOMA

Perioperative NACT for GBC
TMH protocol
Adjuvant chemo:
- **ESPAC 3** for resected periampullary tumors: Gemcitabine versus 5-FU versus Observation. So for resected cholangiocarcinoma, no increase in OS seen.
- **BCAT:** Adjuvant gemcitabine.
- **PRODIGE-12/ACCORD-18:** Adjuvant GEMOX.
BOTH FAILED to show improvement in PFS/OS.

BILCAP: Adjuvant 6 months of capecitabine showed increase in OS in per-protocol analysis with high safety and tolerability. Hence, recommended as current standard of care by NCCN and ASCO.

Adjuvant CRT for R1+ GBC (High Risk)
SWOG-0809 for adjuvant CRT in High-risk GBC (pT2-4, lymph nodes+ surgical margins+): 4#GEMCAP followed by Cap based RT.
Recommended by NCCN and ASCO as adjuvant therapy for GBC with R1 margins.

Palliative Treatment for Inoperable Disease
ABC02: GEMCIS better than gemcitabine alone in advanced biliary tract cancers.

ABC-12 Study: GEMCIS plus Durvalumab was approved by NICE in Jan 2024 as the first line standard of care for those with inoperable cholangioca or GBC.

***PRODIGE 38-AMEBICA*:** GEMCIS versus mFOLFIRINOX (more toxic). No difference in PFS and OS.

ONGOING TRIALS *for resectable GBC*:
- ***GAIN trial*:** For Perioperative GEMCIS versus upfront surgery in GBC.
- ***POLCAGB*:** For NACRT versus NACT in GBC.
- ***JCOG 1202 (ASCOT)*** trial: Adjuvant S1 versus observation. S1 shows promise.

Index

Page numbers followed by *f* refer to figure, *fc* refer to flowchart and *t* refer to table.

A

Abdomen
  lump in 178
  surgical scars in 37
  rest of 9, 39, 135
Abdominal aortic lymph node 25
Abdominal colectomy 165
Abdominal compartment syndrome 117
Abdominal distension 122, 180
Abdominal examination 9, 38, 57, 118, 133, 148, 167
Abdominal surgery 141
Abscess 137, 146, 174
  fungal 93
  hepatic 181
  splenic 189
Achalasia 5, 6, 19
  cardia 16
Achlorhydria 31
Acid-fast bacillus smear, positive 174
Acute variceal bleed, management of 136
Adalimumab 172
Addiction 150
Adenocarcinoma 188
Adenoma 189
Adenomatous polyposis coli 146
Adequate hydration 4
Adjuvant gemcitabine 212
Adrenal mass 189
Adrenal retroperitoneum 179
Advanced unresectable esophageal malignancy, history of 7
Adventitious sounds 10
Albumin infusion 47
Alcoholic hepatitis 124
Alkali consumption 40
Alveolar echinococcosis 184
  classification of 185, 185*t*
Amebic liver abscess 93
Ampullary tumors 120
Anastomosis 103
Anemia 122, 189
Ankylosing spondylitis 165, 167

Anomalous pancreaticobiliary ductal junction 79
Anorectal manometry 150
Anorexia 124
Antibiotic use, history of long-term 166
Aorta 51
Appendectomy, history of 165
Appendix 179
Appetite 150
  loss of 7, 11, 55, 146, 165
Arterial pseudoaneurysms 123
Arthritis 165, 167
Ascending colon 178
  cancer, surgery for 154
Ascites 180
Aspiration pneumonitis, history of 7
Asthma, bronchial 37
Atezolizumab 212
Atrophy hypertrophy complex 79
Azathioprine 170
Azygos 51

B

Back pain 180
  history of 7
Balloon expulsion test 150
Bevacizumab 206, 212
Bile duct 187
  injury 107, 108
Bile leakage after hepatobiliary and pancreatic surgery, grading of 100, 100*t*
Bile refeeding 112
Biliary cirrhosis
  primary 109
  secondary 110
Biliary colic 59, 117
Biliary hamartoma 181
Biliary obstruction, relieves 128
Biliary parasites 120
Biliary stone disease 53
Biliary stricture, benign 109, 116, 118
Bilious vomiting 47
Biliovascular injury, complex 111

Biloma 181, 187
Biopsy 7, 70
  deeper 15
Bleeding per rectum, history of 145
Blood
  clots, presence of 164
  loss, large volume 103
  transfusion 145
  urea nitrogen 99
Bloody stools, frequency of 168
Blunt abdominal trauma 117
Bone
  marrow, compensatory hyperplasia of 132
  painful 117
Bony pain 180
Borderline resectable
  disease 68
  pancreatic cancer 68
Bornman-Terblanche-Blumgart syndrome 180
Botox injection 22
Bowel bladder habits 150
Bowel injury 108
Bowel ischemia 117
Bowel sounds
  auscultate for 39, 58, 119, 168
  reduced 39
Breath, shortness of 11
Brittle diabetes 128
Budesonide 165
Bursectomy 26

C

Cabozantinib 78
Calcineurin inhibitor 169
Calcium 122
  gluconate 191
Cancer 16, 145, 171, 172
  cachexia 192
  uncinate process 69
Capecitabine 73
Carcinoembryonic antigen 65
Carcinoids 32
Cardiovascular diseases 122
Cecum 178
  surgery for 154
Celiac disease 122
Celiac plexus block 126
Cervical
  anastomosis 17
  wound inflammation 49
Chemotherapy
  administration of 7
  perioperative 28
  role of 155

Chest
  pain 36
  disorder 6
  surgical scars in 37
Chicago classification 21*fc*
Child's classification 135*t*
Child-Turcotte-Pugh classification 135
Choking, history of 7
Cholangiocarcinoma 90, 212
Cholangitis 54, 59, 113, 124
  uncontrolled 68
Cholecystectomy 80, 82, 117, 120
Cholecystitis 59, 107
Choledochoduodenostomy 129
Choledochojejunostomy 129
Choledocholithiasis 107, 123
  management of 82
Cholelithiasis 123
Cholestasis 98
Chromoendoscopy, use of 15
Chronic liver disease 54, 107, 135, 137
  signs of 138
  stigmata of 56, 133
Chronic obstructive pulmonary disease 37
Chyle leak 48, 50, 104
  grades 104*t*
  management of 50
Ciplox 172
Cirrhosis 98, 138
Clostridium difficile 166
Coagulopathy 68, 97
Colectomy, subtotal 151, 162
Colon
  conduit, types of 45
  injury 108
  splenic flexure of 179
Colon cancer 205
  management principles of 154
Colonic lesion 188
Colonoscopy 150
Colorectal cancer 147, 152, 208
  TNM staging classification for 195*t*
Colorectal liver metastases 158
Colorectal malignancy, primary 151
Colorectal stage grouping 197*t*
Colo-urinary fistula 146
Coronary and triangular ligaments, dissection of 79
Corrosive consumption injury, emergency management of 40
Corrosive injury 35
Corrosive intake, history of 7
Corrosive stricture 6, 16, 20
Cowden syndrome 147
Crohn's disease 122, 166, 171, 172, 208

Montreal classification for 171
Cruveilhier–Baumgarten sign 135
Cryoablation 73
Cyanosis 118, 166
Cyclosporine 170
Cyst 189
  choledochal 53, 79, 80, 120, 181
  fluid
    biochemical analysis of 65
    glucose 65
  parasitic 189
  pelvic 95
  simple 181
  splenic 189
  true 189
  walls, enhancing 93
Cystic echinococcosis 181
  classification of 182t
Cystic fibrosis 123
Cystic lesions of pancreas 65, 66t
Cystic liver lesion 63, 93
Cystic metastases 93, 181
Cystic pancreatic
  endocrine neoplasm 66
  lesions, fluid analysis of 66
Cystobiliary communication 184

D

Deep vein thrombosis 4
Dehydration, causes 112
Descending colon cancer, surgery for 155
Diabetes
  history of recent onset 55
  mellitus 98
  recent onset of 59
Diarrhea 31
  infective 166
  large bowel 164
  watery 164
Distended gallbladder 57
Drainage procedures 126
Dry cough 180
Duodenal injury repair 52
Duodenal periampullary 59
Duodenal stenosis 123
Duodenum, inflammatory narrowing of 115
Durvalumab 212
Dyselectrolytemia 191
Dyspepsia 10
  history of 10
Dysphagia 5, 7, 35
  complete 37
  diagnosis of malignant 7
  history of 5, 6
  transfer 5

E

Early enteral nutrition 170
Early satiety, history of 11
Ebstein fever 189
Echinococcal cyst, ultrasonography
  classification of 182t
Ectopic kidney 179
Ectopic varices 140
Electrolytes 62, 191
Empyema 188
Endocarditis, infectious 137
Endocrine 127
Endoscopic cystogastrostomy 116
Endoscopic dilatation 22
  principles of 41
Endoscopic procedure, history of 116
Endoscopic removal 31
Endoscopic steroid 22
Endoscopic ultrasound 15
Endoscopic vacuum therapy 49
Endoscopic variceal control 141
Endoscopically refractory variceal bleed 140
Endotoxemia 112
Epigastric pain 36, 59
Epigastrium 178
Erectile dysfunction 176
Erythema nodosum 167
Erythrocyte sedimentation rate 169
Esophageal adenoca 18
  distal 18
Esophageal cancer 5
Esophageal dysphagia 5
Esophageal perforation, management of 47
Esophageal spasm, distal 6
Esophageal stricture 7, 22, 41
Esophageal transection 141
Esophageal tumor 194
Esophageal varices, classification for grading
  of 139t
Esophagectomy
  transhiatal 17, 18
  transthoracic 17
Esophagitis 6
Esophagocele 42
Esophagogastric junction 21
Esophagus 5, 16, 193t
  cancer 202
  case 5
  transection 142
Essential fatty acids 122
Everolimus 211
Exocrine insufficiency, severe 128
Extrahepatic bile duct, distal 200t
Extrahepatic portal vein obstruction 135, 137

Index

Eyes
  examination of 167
  watery 165

F

Familial adenomatous polyposis 146
Familial pancreatitis 120
Fatigue 11, 31, 165
  history of 145
Fecal fat absorption, coefficient of 123
Fecaluria, history of 146
Feeding jejunostomy 9, 36
  tube in situ 37
Felty syndrome 189
Fever 165, 169
  history of 54, 146
Fibrolamellar hepatocellular carcinoma 92
Fibrosis 98
Fissure 149, 168
  in Ano, indicative of 146
Fistula
  external 174
  in Ano, external opening of 149, 168
  internal 174
  risk score 102t
  risk zones 102t
  simple 172
Fluid 191
Focal nodular hyperplasia 179
Folic acid 122
Formal pancreatic resection 71
Free fluid, tests for 9, 39, 119, 135, 149, 168
Frey's procedure 128
Functional lumen imaging probe 21
Fundal varices 142
Fungal disease 20

G

Gallbladder 178, 188
  cancer 59, 65, 107, 197t, 212
    management 85
  demand biopsy of 112
  palpable 59
Gallstone 189
  disease 86
Gastrectomy 23
  distal 24
  non-standard 23
  proximal 24
  selection of 24
  total 24
Gastric adenocarcinoma 10
Gastric cancer 23, 204, 208
Gastric distensibility, reduced 11

Gastric distention 101
Gastric emptying
  delayed 101
  mechanical causes of abnormal 101
Gastric lesion 188
  distal 11
Gastric lymphomas, treatment of 29
Gastric neuroendocrine
  neoplasm 32t
  tumors 32
Gastric outlet obstruction 4, 10, 11
Gastric peristalsis, visible 12, 38
Gastric strictures, grade 42
Gastric surgery, types of 23
Gastric tumor 12
Gastric vein, preserve left 141
Gastroesophageal junction cancer 5, 202, 204
Gastroesophageal reflux disease 6
  history of long-standing 7
Gastroesophageal varices, Sarin classification of 139t
Gastrointestinal bleed 180
Gastrointestinal cancers, TNM staging of 193
Gastrointestinal lymphoma 28, 28t
Gastrointestinal stromal tumor 30
Gastrojejunostomy 23
Gaucher and Niemann–Pick disease 189
Gene mutation 146
Genitalia, examine 38, 57, 118, 148, 167
Genitals, examine 39, 58, 119, 135, 148, 167
GEP-neuroendocrine neoplasms,
  classification of 31t, 70t
Glucose 191
Groin hernial sites 38, 57, 118, 148, 167

H

Harris–Benedict equation 192
Hassabs surgery 142
Head mass 119
  malignant 115, 116
Heartburn 7
Helicobacter pylori 30
  treatment 30
Hemangioma, large 180
Hematemesis 36, 136
  history of 7, 11, 55
Hematoma 181
Hemodynamic instability 117
Hemoglobin 169
Hemogram 61
Hemoptysis 180
Hemorrhage 54
  early 102
  pancreatic 117

postoperative 100
postpancreatectomy 102, 104
severe 104
Hemorrhoidal artery, superior 155
Hepatic ablation 72
Hepatic adenoma 179
Hepatic artery embolization 73
Hepatic artery
  left 111
  right 111
Hepatic cyst, simple 186
Hepatic cystic metastasis 187
Hepatic debulking 72
Hepatic duct, common 108
Hepatic encephalopathy 180
Hepatic flexure colon cancer, surgery for 154
Hepatic hemangioma 180
Hepatic metastasis 181
Hepatic veins 138
Hepatic venous outflow tract obstruction 97
Hepatitis
  B 98
  C 98
Hepatocellular carcinoma 75, 98, 180, 198*t*
Hepatoduodenal ligament, skeletonization of 100
Hepatopancreatobiliary 53, 61, 65, 85, 91, 97
  cancers, TNM staging of 193
Hepatopancreatoduodenectomy 75
Hepatopulmonary syndrome 142
Hepatorenal syndrome 180
Hepatotomy 114
Hereditary 120
  diffuse gastric cancer 11
  nonpolyposis colorectal cancer 147
  spherocytosis 189
Hiatus hernia 20
Hoarseness of voice, history of 7
Hodgkin's lymphoma 189
Hydatid cyst 93, 181, 184, 189
  management of 184
Hypercalcemia 120
Hypercontractile esophagus 6
Hypergastrinemia 31
Hyperkalemia 191
Hypernatremia 191
Hyperperistaltic bowel sounds 149, 168
Hyperplasia of neuroendocrine cells 31
Hypersplenism, history to suggest 131
Hypertriglyceridemia 120
Hypoalbuminemia 119
Hypogastric plexus, inferior 176
Hypokalemia 112, 191
Hyponatremia 112, 191
Hypotension 103
Hypovolemic shock 103

I

Icterus 118, 180
Idiopathic thrombocytopenic purpura 189
Ileostomy 167
Illness, history of presenting 149
Imatinib 31
Inflammatory bowel disease 164
Inflammatory collection 49
Inflammatory complications 125
Inflammatory edema
  acute attack 116, 123
  chronic attack 116
Inflammatory syndrome 180
Infliximab 208
Insulin 128, 191
Integrated relaxation pressure 21
Intensive care unit 104
  admission, history of 116
Intersphincteric fistula tract, ligation of 172
Intestinal obstruction, subacute 168
Intestinal tuberculosis 164, 172
Intra-abdominal infection 100
Intrabolus pressurization 21
Intracranial pressure 99
Intractable pain 125
Intraductal-papillary mucinous neoplasm 66, 187
Intrahepatic cholangiocarcinoma 92, 199*t*
Intraoperative cholangiogram 129
Iridocyclitis 165, 167
Iron deficiency anemia 16
Isolated corrosive gastric strictures 43
  classification 43*t*
Izbicki procedure 129

J

Janus kinase inhibitor 170
Jaundice 165, 180, 189
  causes of 123
  duration of 53
  early 111
  hydration for 112
  late 109
  malignant surgical obstructive 53
  nature of 53
  obstructive 118
  onset of 53
  sudden onset 53
  surgical obstructive 4, 61
  waxing 59
Jejunogastric intussusception 26
Jejunum, situations for 45
Joint 167
  pain, history of 165

Junctional cancer, management of 25
Juvenile polyposis syndrome 147

K

Kala-azar 189
Kasabach–Merritt syndrome 180
Kenawy sign 135
Kidney
  function tests 61
  lower pole 179
  right 178
Kirsten rat sarcoma 66
  viral oncogene homolog 66

L

Laparoscopic cholecystectomy 112
Large cell neuroendocrine carcinoma 31, 70
Left lower quadrant 167, 179
Left upper quadrant 179
  pain, history of sudden onset 131
Leukemia 189
Leukocytosis 49
Lillys technique 81
Lipase 124
Liver 39, 57, 78, 91, 134, 148, 167, 178
  cell failure 180
  cystic primaries, malignant 187
  directed therapy 73
  disease, etiology of 138
  dullness, upper border of 39 58, 119, 135, 148, 168
  function tests 61
  histology 138
  left lobe of 178
  lesions 179
  metastasis 167
    percutaneous ablation of 73
    unresectable 159, 160
  mucinous
    cystic neoplasm of 187
    neoplasms of 186
  primary 93
  secondaries 94
  space occupying lesion 93
  surface 79
Localized gastric nets, management of 31
Loss of weight, history of 7, 11, 55, 146
Low anterior resection syndrome 162
Lower esophageal
  sphincter 21
  webs 20
Low-trauma fractures 122
Lugano and Paris staging systems 28t
Lugano staging system 28, 29

Lung
  disease 98
  metastasis 180
Luschka leak, ducts of 108
Lymph node 196
  dissection 24
    indications for 25
Lymphadenopathy, localized 118, 166
Lymphangioscintigraphy 50
Lymphocytes 50
Lymphoma 188, 189
Lymphorrhea 48
Lynch syndrome 146, 151

M

Magnesium 122
Main-duct intraductal papillary mucinous neoplasm 67
Malabsorption 112
Malaria 189
Malignancy 189
Malnutrition 98
Massive splenomegaly 138
Mediastinal widening 20
Melena, history of 7, 11, 55
Mercaptopurine 170
Mesalamine 165
Mesenteric venous lymph node, superior 25
Metabolic acidosis 112
Metastasis 189
Metastatic disease 72
  history of 7, 11, 55, 146
Metastatic gastric
  cancer 23
  nets, management of 32
Metastatic gastrointestinal stromal tumor 31
mFOLFIRINOX 209, 210
  regimen 210
Microlithiasis 120
Micrometastases 196
Microsatellite instability 147
Microwave ablation 73
Midgut neuroendocrine tumors 211
Minimal hepatic encephalopathy 142
Mirizzi's syndrome 109
Mitotic ratea 31, 70
Mixed neuroendocrine non-neuroendocrine neoplasm 31, 70
Mononucleosis, infectious 137
Motility disorder 6
Movement with respiration 57, 58, 119, 134
Mucinous cystic neoplasm 65, 66, 181
Mucocele 188
Mucosal lesions 118
Multicystic appearance 93

Multidisciplinary tumor board 4
Multiple endoscopic interventions, history of 7
Multiple intrahepatic strictures 80
Mutilineage peripheral cytopenias 132

N

Nasogastric tube 36, 101, 103
Nasojejunal tube placement 36
Native esophageal dilatation 42
Nausea 31, 55
Neck
  examination of 38
  inflammation, symptomatic with 49
  surgical scars in 37
Necrotic lymph node 174
Necrotizing pancreatitis, onfected 121
Neuroendocrine
  carcinoma 31, 70
  liver metastasis 78
    frilling classification of 33f
    management of 33t
  neoplasm 31, 70, 210
    liver metastases 33
  tumor 31, 70
Neutropenia 189
Night sweats 189
Nishi classification 26fc
Nissen fundoplication 142
Nonalcoholic steatohepatitis 98
Non-cirrhotic portal hypertension 131
  surgery for 142
  types of surgeries for 141
Non-curative surgery 23
Nonpancreatic causes 122

O

Obesity 98
Obstructive jaundice, causes of 53
Octreotide 211
Oddi dysfunction, sphincter of 120
Odynophagia 35
Oligometastatic gastric cancer, management of 27
Oliguria 103
Omental lesion 189
Omentectomy 26
Ono's sign 7
Oral anticoagulants, stop newer direct 4
Oral cavity, examination of 9, 38, 118, 166
Oriental cholangiohepatitis 79
Original Sugiura-Futugava surgery 141
Osteopenia 122
Osteoporosis 122

P

Pain, history of 10, 53
Palliative chemotherapy 90
Palliative gastrectomy 23
Palliative surgery 23
Pallor 118
Palpable lump 12
Palpate groin hernia sites 39, 58, 119, 135, 148, 167
Palpation 10
Pancreas 94, 201t, 208
  body of 178
  cancer, head of 59, 68
  divisum 120
  head 178
    lymph node, posterior 25
  tail of 179
Pancreatectomy, total 128
Pancreatic adenoca 94
Pancreatic body 69, 71
Pancreatic cancer 55, 208
Pancreatic capsule, posterior 68
Pancreatic cystic neoplasms 94
Pancreatic duct
  adenocarcinoma 68
  stones 116
  undilated 129
Pancreatic enzyme 122
  replacement therapy 122
Pancreatic fistula 118
  postoperative 101
Pancreatic head 69
Pancreatic lesion 189
Pancreatic necrosis, infected 117, 118
Pancreatic neoplasms 189
Pancreatic net 94
Pancreatic neuroendocrine tumor 70
Pancreatic parenchyma 127, 129
Pancreatic protocol CT 94
Pancreatic stent, preoperative placement of 127
Pancreatic surgery 100, 101t
Pancreaticobiliary malignancies, support diagnosis of 63
Pancreaticoduodenectomy 72
Pancreaticojejunostomy, lateral 126
Pancreatitis
  chronic 59, 115-117, 122
  complications of chronic 123
  recurrent acute 120
  surgery for chronic 129
  types of surgery for chronic 126
Pancreatobiliary secretions 191
Pancreatobiliary tumors 120
Panesophageal pressurization 21

Papilla, tumor of 59
Parenchyma 129
  injury 138
  loss of 127, 128
Parenteral nutrition, total 104
Paris staging system 28, 29
Penetrating disease, pathophysiology of 172
Peptic etiology 16
Peptic stricture 6, 20
Peptic ulcer disease 11
Peptide receptor radionuclide therapy 73
Percutaneous catheter drainage, history of 116
Periampullary cancer 55
Periampullary lesion 126
Perianal abscess 149, 168
  and fistulae 172
Perianal pain, history of 146
Perihilar cholangiocarcinoma 74, 107, 109, 199*t*
Peri-stomal hernia 167
Peritoneal reflection, level of 155
Per-oral endoscopic myotomy 20
Per-rectal examination 39, 58, 119
  proforma 10, 149, 168
Persistent ileus 51
Peutz–Jeghers syndrome 147
Pharyngoesophageal corrosive strictures classification 42*t*
Pheochromocytoma 189
Phlegmon 174
Pleural effusion 39, 180
Polycystic liver disease 181, 186
Polyposis 151
Poor nutritional status 68
Portal cavernoma
  cholangiopathy 138, 140
  presence of 138
Portal hypertension 135, 137, 189
  evidence of 138
Post-cholecystectomy 86
Post-embolization syndrome, management of 73
Post-ERCP pancreatitis 105
Post-esophagectomy complications 47
Post-gastrojejunostomy 51
Posthepatectomy complications 97
Posthepatectomy hemorrhage 97
  severity grading of 97*t*
Posthepatectomy liver failure 98, 99
  grading of 99*t*
Postneoadjuvant therapy 63
Postpancreatectomy acute pancreatitis 104
Post-pancreatic resection complications 101
Postprandial fullness, history of 11

Postprandial upper abdominal heaviness, history of 55
Postural dizziness, history of 11, 55, 145
Postural modulation, history of 6
Pouch of Douglas 10, 58, 119
Preanesthesia 3
Prednisolone 170
Primary tumor 195, 198
  resection 72
Proctocolectomy, total 165
Prokinetics, use of 101
Prophylaxis, primary 140
Proton-pump inhibitors 70
Pruritus 107
  history of 116
  presence of 165
  severe 68
Pseudoachalasia 20
Pseudoaneurysm 95, 103
Pseudocyst 66, 115 116, 118, 123, 129, 189
  complications of 123
Pseudomembranous colitis 166
Psychic moans 117
Pulmonary diseases, history of 37
Pulmonary morbidity, lesser 19
Pulse 169
Pyloroplasty 141, 142
Pylorus-preserving gastrectomy 24
Pyoderma gangrenosum 167
Pyogenic cholangitis, recurrent 109
Pyogenic liver abscess 93

Q

Quality of life 68

R

Radiation exposure, history of 166
Radical antegrade modular pancreatosplenectomy 68
Radio-frequency ablation 73
Ramucirumab 78
Rapid drink challenge 21
Rectal cancer 153, 157, 206
  management principles of 155
  surgery for 156
Rectal prolapse 145, 149
  clinical case of 149
  management of 150
Regional lymph nodes 198
Regorafenib 78
Regurgitation 7
  history of 6
Relaparotomy 103
Renal cysts, multiple 186

Renal dysfunction 112
Renal insufficiency 68, 98
Renal mass 189
Renal stones 117
Resectable liver metastases 160
Resectable pancreas cancer 68
Resected invasive cancer 68
Respiratory examination 10, 39, 119
Retroperitoneal debridement, video-assisted 116
Retroperitoneal mass 189
Retroperitoneum 178, 179
Rheumatoid arthritis 189
Rhonchi 39
Right lower quadrant 167, 178
Right posterior sectoral duct 108
Right upper quadrant 167, 178
Roux-en-Y hepaticojejunostomy 80
Rule out carcinoma 20
Ryles tube, persistent high output 51

S

Saliva, drooling of 36
Sarcoidosis 189
Schatzki ring 20
Schnelldorfer classification 186, 186*t*
Sclerosing cholangitis, primary 109, 165-167
Secretin-Cerulein test 122
Secretin-Pancreozymin test 122
Sectoral duct
    ligation of right posterior 108
    right anterior 114
Sensorium, altered 180
Sepsis 98
    controlled 50
    severe 49, 50
Seroma 181
Serous cystic neoplasm 66, 67
Serum
    amylase 124
    chromogranin 70
Sexual development 140
Short course radiotherapy 206
Shortness of breath, history of 145
Shunt, selective 141
Sideropenic dysphagia 16
Sigmoid cancer 155
Sigmoid colectomy 155
Sigmoid colon 179
    cancer, surgery for 155
Sigmoidostomy 167
Single lumen 167
Sinus 149, 168
    visible 118
Sister Mary Joseph nodule 9, 12

Skin
    excoriation 108, 167
    for scratch marks, examination of 118
    lesions 167
        history of 165
Sleep 150
Small bowel diarrhea 164
Small cell neuroendocrine carcinoma 31, 70
Smoking, history of 11, 166
Soft brown earthy stones 79
Solid liver lesion 62
    benign 91
    malignant 92
Solid pseudopapillary neoplasm 66
Somatostatin
    analogs, long-acting 73
    receptors 71
Sorafenib 212
Spillage 184
Spleen 39, 58, 148, 167, 179
    enlarged 133
Splenectomy 141, 142
Splenic dullness, length of 135
Splenic flexure colon cancer, surgery for 155
Splenic infarct 137
    indicative of 131
Splenic vein thrombosis 123
Squamous cell carcinoma 16
Standard gastrectomy 23
Stanley criteria 125
Steatohepatitis, chemotherapy-associated 98
Steatorrhea 127
Steatosis 98
Steroid refractory 170
STK11 gene mutation 147
Stomach 23, 142, 178, 191, 194*t*
    cancer, proximal 5, 20
    cases 5
    distal 178
    left kidney 179
    proximal half of 142
Stomal stenosis 26
Stools
    color of 54
    maroon colored 145
Storage disorders 189
Stress ulcer 103
Stridor 36
Sudden gripping band, history of 6
Sunken stoma 167
Supraclavicular lymph node, left 118
Supradiaphragmatic mass ligation 51
Surgery, indications for 41, 174
Surgical resection 67
Suspicious mass lesion 79

Synchronous colorectal liver metastases
 management 159
Syncope 11
 history of 145

T

Tachycardia 103
Tacrolimus 169
Tactile vocal fremitus 39
Tail cancer 69
Temozolomide 73, 211
Tenderness 58, 119
Terlipressin 47
Terminal ileum 178
Therapeutic antitubercular trial 174
Therapeutic consequence 103, 104
Thiamine 122
Thoracic anastomosis 17
Thoracic duct injury 48
Thoracoscopic splanchnicectomy 126
Thoracotomy, right posterolateral 48
Thrombocytopenia 98
 severe 140
Timed barium esophagram 21
Tofacitinib 170
Total hepatic vascular exclusion 78
Toxic megacolon 170, 172
 Jalan's criteria for 170
Trachea central 39
Tracheobronchial tear during transhiatal
 esophagectomy, management of 48
Tracheoesophageal fistula 7
Traditional hilar dissection 78
Transverse colon 178
 cancer, surgery for 155
Transverse colostomy 167
Traube's space 135
Tremelimumab 212
Triglycerides 50
Troublesome esophagogastric reflux 18
Tumor
 cells 196
 deposits 196
 extension 28, 29
 high-grade 72
 small 71
Tylosis palmaris et plantaris 16
Typhoid 137, 189
Tyrosine kinase inhibitor 30, 31
 sunitinib 73

U

Ulcerative colitis 168
 management of acute severe 170

Montreal classification for 169
severity of 168
steroid-dependent 170
steroid-refractory 169
treatment of mild-to-moderate 169
Umbilical nodule 9, 12
Undescended testis tubo-ovarian structures 179
Upper abdominal fullness 12
Upper gastrointestinal
 corrosive injury 35
 ward 47
Urine output 99
 reduced 180

V

Vagotomy 141
Variceal bleed 180
 medical management of 47
Variceal rebleeding 136
Vedolizumab 169
Vertebral metastasis 180
Viral disease 20
Vitamin
 A, fat-soluble 122
 D 54
  fat-soluble 122
  deficiency, fat soluble 54, 112
 E 54
  fat-soluble 122
 K 4, 54
  fat-soluble 122
Voice, hoarseness of 36
Voluminous nonbilious vomiting 55
Vomiting 31, 101
 history of 11
von Meyenburg complex 181

W

Waning jaundice 59
Warfarin 4
Weight loss, history of 165
Wheeze 39
Whipple 128

X

Xanthogranulomatous cholecystitis 188

Z

Zargar classification 36*t*
Zinc 122
Zollinger–Ellison syndrome 32, 122